INFLUENCE OF MEDIA ON PUBLIC HEALTH

Solutions to Healthcare Surveillance Issues in Nigeria, Africa and Around the World

written by

Mary-Jane Ilozor

STORYMAKERS, Inc.

Published in 2022 by

STORYMAKERS, INC.
P.O. Box 91338
Houston, Texas 77291-1338
www.storymakersinc.com

ISBN: 978-0-9888079-9-0

Printed in the United States of America

TABLE OF CONTENTS

ACKNOWLEDGEMENT   xi

FOREWORD

**The Hon. Nze Ogochukwu Vincent
Okpala, MD.**   xiii
COMMISSIONER FOR HEALTH, ANAMBRA STATE,
NIGERIA

Vincent I. Maduka   xv
RETIRED DIRECTOR-GENERAL, NIGERIAN
TELEVISION AUTHORITY (NTA)
FORMER SENIOR FELLOW, PAN-ATLANTIC
UNIVERSITY, LAGOS, NIGERIA

Emeka Onodugo   xix
BUSINESS MANAGER, CHI PHARMACEUTICALS LTD.

INTRODUCTION   1

History of Nigerian Print Media   5

CHAPTER ONE **Examination of Nigerian Print
Media on Its Healthcare
Surveillance Role**

Overview   9

Factors Responsible for Content Imbalance   19

- ADVERTISING DEGRADES DELIVERY OF HEALTHCARE CONTENT
- ENTERTAINMENT MORE POPULAR THAN HEALTHCARE INFORMATION
- RELIGION DIVERTS ATTENTION FROM VALID HEALTHCARE ISSUES
- SUPERNATURAL INFORMATION PERVADES MEDIA
- OVERUSE OF PUBLIC ALERTS DIMINISHES ATTENTION TO HEALTHCARE ISSUES
- POLITICS PREEMPTS IMPORTANT HEALTHCARE INFORMATION

Recommendations   33

- USE OF ADVERTISEMENTS TO ADDRESS HEALTHCARE
- BALANCING OF HEALTHCARE CONTENT ADVISED
- HEALTHCARE INFORMATION PROMOTION ON PRINT ICT MEDIA AND PAPER PRINT MEDIA
- CONSISTENCY
- SALARY OF HEALTHCARE JOURNALISTS
- MORE HEALTHCARE PRINT MEDIA COMPANIES, JOURNALISTS, SCIENCE, AND MEDICALS REQUIRED
- PROFESSIONAL JOURNALISTS ON HEALTHCARE SURVEILLANCE
- CITIZEN JOURNALISM ON PRINT DIGITAL MEDIA IMPROVING HEALTHCARE
- PARTNERSHIPS BETWEEN JOURNALISTS AND HEALTHCARE PROFESSIONALS IN TRAINING JOURNALISTS
- TRAINING AND AWARDING OF JOURNALISTS FOR HEALTHCARE COVERAGE
- PRINT ICT-BASED MEDIA ON HEALTHCARE

CHAPTER TWO   **Influence of Media Campaign on Positive Healthcare Behavior Change and Social Transformation**

Overview   43

Social Problems Targeted with Media Campaigns   51

- TOBACCO USE
- ALCOHOL USE
- LACK OF PHYSICAL ACTIVITY
- POOR NUTRITION
- CARDIOVASCULAR DISEASE PREVENTION
- BIRTH RATE REDUCTION
- HIV INFECTION PREVENTION
- CERVICAL CANCER SCREENING AND PREVENTION
- BREAST CANCER SCREENING AND PREVENTION
- BOWEL CANCER SCREENING AND PREVENTION
- SKIN CANCER PREVENTION
- IMPROVED IMMUNIZATION
- DIARRHOEAL DISEASE PREVENTION
- INCREASED BREASTFEEDING
- IMPROVED ROAD SAFETY
- INCREASED ORGAN DONATION
- IMPROVED MENTAL HEALTH AND REDUCED VIOLENCE AND CHILD MALTREATMENT
- IMPROVED PREHOSPITAL RESPONSE TIMES FOR POTENTIAL HEART ATTACK SYMPTOMS

Recommendations   85

- GOVERNMENT AGENCIES IN CONJUNCTION WITH HEALTH ORGANIZATIONS AND OTHER POLICY MAKING BODIES

- REGULATIONS ON SOCIAL MEDIA TO REDUCE MISGUIDANCE, SOCIAL NORMS, AND BELIEFS AFFECTING THE FUNCTIONALITIES OF MEDIA CAMPAIGN
- INDIRECT INFUSED CAMPAIGNS
- FUNDING
- PROVISION OF HEALTH CENTERS AND FACILITIES
- REGULATING COMPETING INFLUENCES AFFECTING HEALTHCARE MEDIA CAMPAIGNS
- MULTISECTORIAL AND INTERSECTORAL COLLABORATION
- PROPER ENVIRONMENT FOR FITNESS AND PHYSICAL HEALTH PROGRAMS
- PRIVATE SECTOR PARTICIPATION IN MEDIA CAMPAIGNS
- RESEARCHERS AND WELL-INFORMED CAMPAIGN PLANNERS
- IDENTIFYING THE TARGET AUDIENCE
- USE OF TESTIMONIALS FOR ATTRACTIVE CAMPAIGNS

CHAPTER THREE **Media and Journalists Role of Surveillance in Healthcare Communication**

Overview   99

Basic Roles of Healthcare Journalists and Problems Identified   110

- INFORM AND EDUCATE THE PUBLIC ON HEALTH AWARENESS AND THE ENVIRONMENT
- POLICY AND SOCIAL INFLUENCERS ON HEALTH ISSUES
- HEALTH INFORMATION AND CAMPAIGN PROMOTION THROUGH OTHER DEPARTMENTS UNDER MEDIA

- IDENTIFYING THE KEY STAKEHOLDERS IN HEALTHCARE AND ESTABLISHING A PROFESSIONAL RELATIONSHIP
- UNDERSTANDING THE COMPLEXITY OF HEALTHCARE SYSTEM AND IMPROVING TRANSFORMATIONAL METHODOLOGIES
- CAPACITY BUILDING BY EMPOWERING NEW HEALTHCARE JOURNALISTS
- ATTENDING HEALTH CONFERENCES AND COORDINATING HEALTHCARE CAMPAIGNS

Recommendations   123

- INVESTIGATIVE JOURNALISM TO BE MONITORED IN HEALTHCARE
- STRATEGIC PLANS BY THE MEDIA ARE NEEDED FOR STAGE-MANAGING NEGATIVE RESPONSES ON HEALTH REPORTS
- ALL MEDIA ACTIVITIES TO FOLLOW MEDIA PROCEDURES AND BE ACCOUNTABLE
- GATEKEEPING IN MEDIA NEEDS ACTIVATION AND IMPROVEMENT
- POSITIONING OF MEDIA INSTITUTIONS AS WATCHDOGS AND FOURTH ESTATE OF THE REALM ON HEALTH CASES
- INTEGRATION OF HEALTHCARE COMMUNICATION ACROSS ALL SECTORS BY ENCOURAGING THE NEW INITIATIVES EHEALTH AND MHEALTH

ABOUT THE AUTHOR   133

GLOSSARY   135

REFERENCES   137

ACKNOWLEDGEMENT

Special appreciation to God and the heavenly Kingdom, for seeing me through this project, I forever remain thankful.

Gratitude to my family and friends for their encouragement and support, my children Danny, Ella, Lora (Oma), and Olivia (Chichi), all Emeka-Ilozor's, my husband Engr. John Chukwuemeka Ilozor for being a part of my life and achievements. All thanks to my Late Dad (Mr. Raphael Sunday C. Muo) and my Mom (Mrs. Joy Ifechinyere Muo) for all their sacrifices raising me with my siblings without doubts of my future attainments in life and nurturing me to become my dream self. God bless your efforts, much love Daddy and Mommy. Thanks to my in-laws, Late Father-in-law, Pa Innocent I. Ilozor, my mother-in-law, Ma Josephine Ilozor.

Thank you, Fred Stawitz and Storymakers, Inc., USA, for believing in me, bringing out the best in me, thus this publication and more to be unleashed. I cannot thank you enough, Fred, for everything. I appreciate you.

I appreciate you Emeka Onodugo, you have always been there, through my career ladder, your continuous advice and countless times of proffering solutions, when issues arise is priceless.

I remain grateful to Engr. Vincent Maduka for all your mentorship since I graduated from Pan-Atlantic University (SMC). You so much understand me and I am thankful to God, having someone humble and caring as you by my side. Thank you, my Prof!

Thank you, Dr. Mike Okolo, Dean of Studies, School of Media and Communications (SMC), Pan-Atlantic University (PAU). I appreciate all your encouraging words. Same goes to Dr. Bel Molokwu, Dr. Felix Ibode, Dr. Isah Momoh, Dr. Sunday Olarunto, Dr. Nweze Ndubisi Nwosu, Dr. Ngozi Okpara, Dr. Anuli, and all SMC, PAU facilitators. Gratitude to my friend and coursemate Temisan Ojabo, and all my FT7 Class of 2015 SMC, PAU Alumni. I appreciate your encouragement.

Thanks to the Hexavians of Eizu Uwaoma and all my friends who enjoy seeing my career blossom.

Thanks to good family-friends like Oliver Enweonwu, Rex Mafiana, and Prince McMishael for your encouraging words. I am grateful.

Thanks to friends like Mr. Wenigha Churchill, Mrs. Lydia Enyidiya Eke, Mrs. Florence Okah-Avae, Mr. Akinola Afolabi, and all my friends at Unilag Radio and TV media. Thanks to Dr. Patrick Oloko, Dr. Okoro of the English Department at Unilag.

Thanks for the prayers and advice of friends like Rev. Fr. Charles Egbon, Rev. Fr. JohnPaul, Rev. Fr. Anthony Fadairo, Msgr. Philip Hoteyin, Emmanuel Chiadi Ndubuisi, Osita Ignatius Odili, Barr. Kehinde Oludare, Emmanuel Effiong, Valentine, and Rose Nwabueze, Dr. Ndubuisi Nwosu, Prof. Dr. Ogedemgbe, Dr. Adegun of Mariam Clinics, and everyone who has been part of my success in any way. I appreciate you all.

I remember my late family-friends, Barr. Christopher Officha, Fidelix N. Onaku for their fatherly advice and nurturing while I was growing up. I know they are celebrating my achievements in heaven. God bless their souls.

And, thanks to my readers. I appreciate you all.

FOREWORD

The Hon. Nze Ogochukwu Vincent Okpala, M.D.

COMMISSIONER FOR HEALTH, ANAMBRA STATE, NIGERIA

Influence of Media on Public Health is a great addition to the armamentarium of the public health practitioner, especially with respect to the management of infodemics. Mary-Jane Ilozor just handed her peers and health policymakers a much-needed tool in dealing with misinformation and disinformation in the age of the reign of social media. The worrisome social media influence on COVID-19 vaccine hesitancy shows that public health experts and members of the fourth estate must work together to achieve a healthy society, and for this group, this book is a must-read!

Vincent I. Maduka

RETIRED DIRECTOR-GENERAL, NIGERIAN TELEVISION AUTHORITY (NTA)
FORMER SENIOR FELLOW, PAN-ATLANTIC UNIVERSITY, LAGOS, NIGERIA

Mary-Jane Ilozor, author of *Influence of Media on Public Health,* is, in all respects, a communicator. The objective of the publication is, essentially, the promotion of healthy living, a matter that should be of common, indeed, mass interest. We are looking at the entire gamut of human well-being: from birth, nay, conception, to birth, and growing up and growing old. As regards health, the required skill and competence would, properly, reside in a health professional or expert, the doctor, nurse, physiotherapist and all the other highly skilled personnel in that industry.

The concern of the reader of this publication is the matter of the good message of healthy living: what to do to prevent poor health and illness and, up to a point, what to do when illness strikes. While these are most vital, what people do not have enough time and knowledge to undertake is what to do in order to keep illness at bay, since most people do not bother about their health until they actually lose it.

Fitness, whether physical or mental, is often neglected by citizens going about their daily lives. Indeed, most people who undertake physical fitness exercise, or controlled dietary practices as deliberate pursuits, are people who are generally enlightened, and who may be described as elitist: often, they are trying to keep trim in figure, lose weight or reduce tummy shape and that sort of thing, usually for looks, but admittedly, also, for good health. The author of the subject publication was, for several years, engaged in producing and participating in physical exercise, gym-type sweat and fat burning endeavors for television broadcasting. Unless undertaken as prescribed by the doctor, this form of promotion of (public) health is essentially middle-class, and is very easily taken up by fashionable women, in particular, and also quite easily dropped, as it is difficult to sustain. Our author is quite experienced in this line of communicating physical exercise.

As regards the prevention of diseases and illness, Mrs. Ilozor is a Communicator and Journalist, and is eminently qualified to dabble, indeed, speak to the public on the media. She holds a Master's degree in English, the official medium of communication in Nigeria, obtained from one of the foremost universities in Nigeria, the University of Lagos. In addition, she has a Master's degree in Communication from the trail-blazing Pan-Atlantic University near Lagos. Often times, the specialists in health matters (as well as in other human issues) are not the best people to explain to the ordinary members of the public, in simple words, what people should know and do in the respective specialized disciplines: it requires a communicator.

The medic may be exasperated that the ordinary Nigerian man or woman rejects the COVID vaccination, for example, something that any sensible person should gratefully embrace. The doctor says, quite simply, take this vaccine, if you don't take it, you will be ill and, probably, die. The journalist, on the other hand, is interested in why that Nigerian rejects the vaccine, and properly seeks to understand in order to be able to convey or communicate the status accurately. The communicator's, or the advertiser's, job is to present the product in a manner that the people, practically, scramble to receive it. For example, having the vaccine could be made to confer a status symbol: the Nigerian loves status and class, it is the professional communicator who is going to exploit this characteristic to be successful, and not so easily the scientist.

The social media may be currently flooded with cynicism, but its reach, popularity, and power cannot be dismissed lightly. Its effectiveness in the promotion of public health, for example, should be appreciated for its numbers and reach, as well as its demography. It takes a trained and involved social media practitioner and communicator to take full advantage of the social media: talks/posts, music and dance, comedy, drama, animation, name it. Our author is at home in both the conventional and the new media, and the reader will benefit immensely from her wealth of exposure.

Emeka Onodugo

BUSINESS MANAGER, CHI PHARMACEUTICALS LTD.

Clearly there is a huge gap in reporting healthcare issues in the media in a developing country like Nigeria and other countries around the world. Mary-Jane Ilozor's ability to have recognized this problem, and her skill in enabling others to understand the implications, is the great achievement of this publication.

Influence of Media in Public Health is a publication which focuses on healthcare prevention provisions and the role of the media in timely reporting from reliable sources. It is aimed at achieving standard media representation and support in tracking some of the challenges of public healthcare situations in Nigeria and the world.

The reader will definitely benefit from the revelations in the publication, pushing the narrative on improving healthy living with knowledge of some basic healthcare updates and practices, if only relevant information is timely promoted in the media for the sake of the poor and vulnerable living in rural communities.

The publication is comprehensive, informative, educative, insightful, and a recommended required reading for media practitioners especially in a developing country like Nigeria. I commend Mary-Jane Ilozor for this initiative and for sharing her experiences and knowledge with others. This book is worth more than its price.

INTRODUCTION

Healthcare communication is everyone's responsibility, but professionally the media, government, healthcare givers or organizations (both international and local) are expected to keep updating the masses on ways of improving good healthy livelihood. To achieve this obligation, there is much dependency on the media as the intermediate institution, between both healthcare institutions/government and the public. Media, as the Fourth Estate of the Realm, has the mobilizing power which is backed with government policies in implementing healthcare provisions and recommendations for preventing pandemic, outbreak, infection, and other forms of diseases.

Influence of Media on Public Health provides solutions to healthcare surveillance issues in Nigeria, Africa and around the world. It is directed towards achieving standard media representation and support in compliance to journalists' obligations in tackling public healthcare. Most references are Nigerian sources and are digested to a simple English language for clarification and easy comprehensibility for all readers, especially the tertiary institutions in media practices, post graduates, and researchers. Media professionals as the major target audience need the reformations recommended in this book for more impacting services while protecting masses' interest in preserving healthy lives.

The focus is on healthcare preventive mechanisms and media's timely reports from reliable sources with accurate data and figures in presentation and professionalism proven, without negligence on equity and equality in healthcare practices. It points at those who doubt the new normal protocols, recommended vaccinations and healthcare related programs like cancer campaigns reaching out to every community without prejudice or negligence on the local communities. The rural communities have been the concern of the negligence in healthcare treatments or disease control and this needs to be resolved quickly to ensure equity in service to humanity. The masses in the rural communities are less informed and most times are being disregarded on some basic healthcare updates and practices. The recommendations on this publication provide solutions to rectifying and resolving most of these issues detected in media practices.

Stakeholders in healthcare and media institutions are parts of the beneficiaries and target audience of this publication, as regards documentation, references and studies. This well-researched book, *Influence of Media on Public Health* provides readers with the fundamentals of improving healthy living with knowledge on the hindrances that could be encountered and solutions in view with recommendations on best practices in all chapters. Every chapter is informative and thoroughly researched with references from online sources that are easy to locate in a click. References and sources are obtained from links, such as the World Health Organization (WHO), other reliable international healthcare organizations, researchers' works, and more.

Some issues regarding the recent COVID-19 pandemic, which has outburst of variants discovered from named Delta and Omicron inspired this publication on healthcare. The disturbing emergence of these variants is one of the reasons for more researches in healthcare, as the masses are listening and patiently waiting for an end to this. The media becomes the hope of stakeholders in healthcare in passing across information for speedy dissemination to the public with accuracy in gathering data and sources. Healthcare stakeholders, like the international and national healthcare organizations the WHO, UN, UNISEF, NAFDAC, pharmaceuticals, medicals, and more are recognized in this research as important bodies that provide updates for the media on health. These organizations provide answers to questions of curious masses on facts and updates regarding healthcare. Such wanderings of the masses are expected to be in circulation with the trust the public embedded on the media institution. Issues concerning new vaccines, like the recent booster jab for COVID-19, recommended drugs, newly mutated variants of COVID-19, and etcetera, are some of the questions weighing the masses down on what the next step is and their part of expectations in compliance to the demands of healthcare professionals/organizations and the government. How do they align with healthcare policies and keep safe with the new norms? When disease detections are discovered, what exactly are they and how does the media manage and reduce publics' panic on strange emerging healthcare issues, with well researched contents availability for all?

Dependency on social media for sources of information is one of issues discussed, which is detected to be harmful most times for news gathering or consumption. The unprofessionalism and non-expertise of ordinary individuals spreading rumors or wrongly displaying communication skills without the rightful knowledge on how information is passed, when to engage people in a serious discourse that deals with life and death cases on healthcare management and other armature ways of sharing news is unacceptable. Fishing out unreliable sources and exposing them to the people, correcting the wrongs and taking the lead are some of the media obligations to tackle. Ignorance is not an excuse and media ought to obstruct the false alarm by exposing these negative impressions of ordinary posters and commentators to obstruct their lies from spreading. Facts gathered by researchers should not be ignored, rather promoting them is very essential for actualizing the purposes of these educative researches for public consumptions. It is recommendable to value researchers' information and partake in disseminating their vital communicable detailed instructions/contents for best health maintenance practices, while motivating the public in complying with recommended norms for disease control in various communities and all around the world.

Solutions to media practices on healthcare presented in this impactful book have great influence in correcting some mistakes and errors discovered which in most cases linger without being checked. Some of these obstacles and healthcare problems discussed in this book take a meticulous fact-finder or detector, to pick and find solutions to them. It is very crucial not to waste time in implementing the corrections and recommendations presented in this publication to achieve the purpose of this work and the motive of brains behind it, for the best media healthcare practice of our generation, the government, healthcare institutions, researchers and more.

Influence of Media on Public Health is highly recommendable and worth the read for any single moment spent reading or gathering sources from it. It is world class documentation for promoting great healthcare. My great hope is that the efforts will be productive with results in changing the media for the best on healthcare journalism, especially in Africa.

History of Nigerian Print Media

The newspaper first appeared in Nigeria on November 23, 1859, when Presbyterian missionary Reverend Henry Townsend published *Iwe Iroyin Fun Awon Ara Egba Ati Yoruba* to serve the Yoruba people, an ethnic group located in Western Nigeria.[1] The name was later shortened to *Iwe Irohin*. "It is the opinion of many that, in contrast to his purported objective, the purpose of Rev. Henry Townsend newspaper was to foster the outreach of Christian religion at the time; it cannot be denied, however, that the *Iwe Irohin* played a very significant role in the history of Nigerian newspaper."[2]

"My objective is to get the people to read and to beget the habit of seeking information by reading," stated the publisher Reverend Henry Townsend.[3] As the founder of the first newspaper in Nigeria, Reverend Henry Townsend expressed what motivated him to publish his newspaper for the Egbas and Yoruba native speakers. *Iwe Irohin* certainly played a very significant role in the history of Nigeria.

Within eight years, *Iwe Irohin* was being published in English and Yoruba. Some of its stories revolve around Abeokuta, a historic region of Nigeria, as well as cotton and cocoa statistics. It is said that the newspaper included advertisements from local firms and government agencies as early as 1860. This publication helped develop the reading habits of Nigerian people and developed their desire to consume news.

The second Nigerian newspaper, the *Anglo-African*, was published by Professor Robert Campbell, a West Indian immigrant, in 1863.[4] This was the first newspaper published in Lagos and was considered to be the "paper of its times" because it was "purposed for African self-improvement through the utilization of Western and African systems of knowledge."[5]

Then, in 1880, Richard Olamiege Beale Blaize with editor Andrew M. Thomas established the *Logos Times and Gold Coast Colony Advertiser*. This was the third newspaper in Nigeria and was mainly concerned with critical issues and matters of the period. "Records even have it that The Lagos Times and Gold Coast Colony Advertiser was actually the first to publicly denounce the extravagance of the colonial government in one of its editions published in 1881. However, the newspaper would go out of circulation on October 24, 1883; only to reappear seven years later with little or no success."[6]

In 1926, what was considered "Nigeria's most enduring and popular newspaper," the *Nigeria Daily Times* was published by the Nigerian Printing and Publishing Company. Ernest Ikoli, editor and head of the renowned King's College in Lagos, Nigeria, established the paper on a "sound commercial basis" while also being "critical of the colonial establishment."[7] Dr. Nnamdi Azikiwe added his voice to the media when he launched the *West African Pilot* in 1937 with the motto: "Show the light and the people will find the way."[8]

In 1949, Chief Obafemi Jeremiah Oyeniyi Awolowo, the son of a Yoruba farmer, founded the *Nigerian Tribune*. Chief Awolowo was a Nigerian nationalist and statesman who played a key role in Nigeria's independence movement. He used the *Nigerian Tribune* "to create a just and egalitarian Nigerian society, re-generate the spirit of altruism and nationalism in Nigerians by promoting the idea of nationhood." This is the oldest surviving newspaper in Nigeria and continues to strive to be the "voice of the voiceless."[9]

Today, Nigeria has numerous newspapers in circulation including *Vanguard, Punch, Nation, The Guardian, Daily Trust, This Day, Sun,* and a host of others.[10] This array of publications offers Nigerians numerous choices of newspapers from which to receive the news in both print and digital distribution platforms. Just to be clear, according to Oxford Reference which is associated with Oxford University Press, *print media* is broadly defined as "any written or pictorial form of communication produced mechanically or electronically using printing, photocopying, or digital methods from which multiple copies can be made through automated processes."[11] This broad definition of print media is applied throughout this publication.

The newspaper was initially an agent of political propaganda and war. Some of the newspapers had issues with the government which led to their sanctioning and restriction from free press. This is why political news has more influence on the print media than others in Nigeria today. "After independence in 1960, the press in Nigeria underwent some major technical and structural changes." Additionally, "the federal government set up a large web offset printing press and took control of the leading dailies that shaped public opinion."[12]

Politicians, corporate executives, and the powerful elites are the greatest consumers of print media in Nigeria. Politics attracts readers, and has from the inception of print media in the country, but access to health news remains a serious concern for readers as well. Unfortunately, the print media being controlled by Nigerian politicians reduces the healthcare content as readers are regularly overfed with political headlines instead of health-related updates.

News content on healthcare or medical issues typically surfaces only when diseases threaten public health on a large scale. This complicates the challenge for the average reader in sorting through other content to find information relevant to a healthy lifestyle. Otherwise, healthcare issues are swept aside along with relevant information provided by doctors and healthcare providers. While the founding fathers of print media in Nigeria pursued the objective of informing, enlightening, educating, and connecting the public with valuable social resources and information relevant to their lives in a full range of areas, the reality of the current situation is that print media falls short, particularly, in the area of timely reporting health issues.

CHAPTER ONE

Examination of Nigerian Print Media on Its Healthcare Surveillance Role

Overview

Media is highly promoted and increasingly influencing the lives of citizens in Nigeria, throughout Africa, and around the world. The media serves as the channel for disseminating information to enlighten consumers by broadcasting news updates which connects individuals to each other and society. Transformation is obtained through the media and it is expected that information from the healthcare sector ought to provide value to the audience, considering its relevance to livelihood.

Healthcare programs enriching the print media field boosts the support of its participants and stakeholders. Such programs help restore trust in health workers, who are devoted to solving health maintenance problems during public healthcare crises.

Journalism is systematic and has developed a vast reach and is more easily accessible than ever before. The future of healthcare journalism and the impact of new media presents a new and exciting terrain to save lives and upgrade healthy living standards in the community. Updating the audience regularly has posed a great challenge to journalists coupled with the social media opportunity in reaching a much wider audience. The new media gives room for users to act upon the content they consume by providing feedbacks to the distributors of the information. Therefore, engaging the audience generally occurs as a result of acknowledging reactions and responses from readers.

Anyone who can read and write is capable of becoming an active participant in journalism, if courageous enough to communicate to the public. The internet availability via smart phones, computer systems, and other communication devices promotes fast responses and cuts the overall costs of such an exchange.

News posting and sharing has become a global affair. Writers reach global audiences and gain feedback from consumer comments within seconds. It is a great opportunity that welcomes greater participation. But health journalism is a serious affair demanding best practices by media professionals and other key participants.

Nigerian print media is like a chameleon; it changes from time to time to suit the current climate. Originally, the print media dominated the communication channel handling various reports and news from numerous sectors of life endeavors. The inability to equitably balance its role in covering essential reports for readers with other activities is questionable. Unfortunately, the print media too often dances to the tune of popular demand, thereby being controlled by the desire of various interest groups or selfish stakeholders, disregarding their fundamental function as the watchdog of the society.

Print media in Nigeria and elsewhere should serve everyone and not only a group of individuals in a particular sector, whose individual agenda usually preempts other media contents including healthcare, while promoting their own message. This minimizes the functionality of journalism at its essence.

Society ought to be presented with their needs, not their wants. A chameleon changes in color based on the domineering color in the background. This description best portrays Nigerian print media in diverting energy to the most popular demand information on a particular news dimension. Thereby, disregarding healthcare information and other important contents of good journalism. This is disturbing and has driven deep in the system causing a troubling content imbalance for readers.

Print-based media "broadly, means any written or pictorial form of communication produced mechanically or electronically using printing, photocopying, or digital methods from which multiple copies can be made through automated processes. It also means any form of 'ink and paper' communication that is not hand-written or hand-typed, including books, circulars, journals, lithographs, memos, magazines, newspapers, pamphlets, and periodicals."[1] This definition provides a clear indication that print media's digital publication is included as a form of print media just like paper publication.

Print ICT-based media has to do with accessing information of publishers online with electronic devices such as mobile phones, desktops, laptops, tablets, iPads, and other similar items that connect to the internet. ICT refers to information and communications technologies. Digital media provides readers with both soft copy/virtual format and hard copy in the form of printed papers, newspapers, magazines, journals, and etc.

The print media existed as one of the traditional media channels before the invention of digital platforms. Its deep effect on the consumers' preferences is currently being accessed. No doubt, the expansion of print media into the realm of ICT presents quite a commendable transformation that can assist journalists in fulfilling their surveillance role on healthcare in particular.

But sadly, health maintenance information is being neglected in journalism and attention is needed by journalists to fulfill their traditional duty as expected. "Health communication is an integral aspect of social marketing and a communication aimed at changing the behaviors of individuals and communities about a certain habit, idea or disease; the media is very important because it provides the platform through which health messages and campaigns are promoted. Health communication is more about prevention than curation, it is therefore the moral obligation and responsibility of media practitioners and experienced communicators to ensure that health maintenance messages and campaigns are successfully executed and must reach the target audience."[2]

Much is expected from journalists, though they face some obstacles limiting their capabilities in fulfilling their roles. Journalists are faced with the dilemma of performing their roles accurately by providing balanced content for all sectors of society with little support. This has been the fundamental issue obstructing media practitioners, especially as related to healthcare. The most sponsored content will be published while information that offers more social benefit is ignored.

Balanced communication on health is not an unimaginable expectation from journalists; it is achievable. It requires knowledge, dedication, selflessness, practical duty obligations, and support from stakeholders including the government as well as international and national medical sectors. Traces of successful healthcare communication was demonstrated during the 2014 Ebola crisis in Nigeria.

This implies that consistency is needed in healthcare information broadcast and publication for solutions to health issues in various communities. "If health communication is a preventive measure of communication, where health messages are disseminated using media technologies and organizations for the purpose of creating awareness about diseases and ailments; then journalists, reporters and their media organizations should treat other diseases which have statistically proven to be more devastating and frequently occur with high mortality rate than Ebola, with a lot of attention by ensuring that frequent health messages and health promotional campaigns are continuously disseminated in the media."[3]

Some extremely dangerous diseases seem to have become more common in Nigeria due to negligence in creating public awareness of the public threat they pose by journalists and has given rise to high death rates in the country. Cholera, yellow fever, chicken pox, and Lassa fever are a few examples of diseases causing deaths, yet little or no attention is directed to them by Nigerian journalists. "There are diseases worse than Ebola that have been present, killing people daily, but do not get the kind of media attention that is needed to promote health education. Cancer, malaria, hypertension, diabetes, obesity and others have killed more people than Ebola; children and women lie helplessly in hospitals and herbal homes, people feed unhealthily, fail to exercise properly and live nonchalant lifestyles that distort their health, yet the media especially in Nigeria ignore these diseases."[4]

Many of the headlines of Nigerian newspapers represent deceitful titles, often in relation to Nigerian politics. Some of these political headlines are seen in the Pulse.[5] Politics tends to rule the press. The front pages of newspapers are saturated with the words and actions of governmental authorities driven by their political ambitions and party aspirations. One wonders what happened to reporting on lifesaving healthcare information?

Nigerians are just as anxious as anyone else in the world to live safe and free from infections and other diseases but the power tussle among

13

politicians leaves little or no publication space for healthcare and disease prevention reports. One hardly sees health content with boldly printed headlines unless there is an active outbreak, epidemic or pandemic. The healthcare sections of Nigerian newspapers only seem to become relevant when health crises arise. Why?

According to Kehinde Gbolahan Somoye in the book *Critical Review of The Management of Healthcare System in Nigeria: Emphasis on Health Workforce*, a "healthcare system can be defined as the aspect of organizing people, resources and institutions which deliver healthcare services to meet the needs of the health of populations targeted."[6] The media plays an essential role; unfortunately, journalists and the media they serve seem to have abdicated one of their fundamental obligations for keeping the public informed on vital issues surrounding health.

Similar to healthcare journalism is medical journalism. "With progression of the technology, medical journalism became a new element of disseminating medical information and help to accelerate the processes of medical changes"[7]

Most people, especially medical workers or stakeholders in the healthcare industry, depend on the release of official reports to keep abreast of relevant health information. "Newspapers and magazines are also often seen as credible or trusted sources."[8] The fact is that newspapers often serve as the official public record for certain public information. Nigerian print media is not an exception. No matter what advances are made in the new digital media regarding the dissemination of valuable public information, print media still remains a relevant repository for such information. The recordkeeping ability of print media in a physical format in libraries, offices or other places backs up data shared on the internet through digital means.

Newspapers, magazines and journals serve the populace even when electricity fails in Nigeria which occurs more frequently in the rural parts of the country. In essence, accessibility via print media is not contingent upon electronic access which means that healthcare information on print media offers a reliable link to lifesaving healthcare cautions and updates regardless of location or access to networks.

The advent of the internet resulted in creation of the popular slogans: "google it," "surf the net," and "check online." Most contemporary readers access information online. As a result, print media as a traditional media is gradually losing its audience to digital media, now the giant of communications channel. Therefore, it is quite reasonable to follow the trend of catching the attention of readers on the digital platform. The internet offers a fast way of reaching out with vital medical information to a majority of the public.

"The growth in digital newspaper readership is in sharp contrast to the trend in physical newspaper circulation."[9] This growth is where journalists should focus attention, providing healthcare information to their readers regarding the benefit of time, location, and the simplicity of communications. Digital print media provides journalists with the latest means to easily disseminate healthcare information. Now, speedy data collection through digital online interviews has opened the door for easy access by journalists to medical personnel with the more recent public health information.

Some healthcare providers are engaging in journalism as freelance journalists by providing valuable public interest information through the internet. They are joining the global digital transformation and filling the gap left by journalists that have not engaged on health matters. Motivated individuals are sharing healthcare information via private publications produced at home or even bulletins disseminated from medical schools, hospitals, and other places of work. Journalism is becoming everyone's responsibility, yet professionalism matters in information delivery of vital healthcare information.

As earlier discussed, the healthcare information availability on the internet provides individuals with access to information from any location through their mobile and stationed electronics devices such as phones, laptops, desktops, iPads, tablets, and etcetera. Facilitated by these devices, social media has become an effective tool for sourcing and disseminating news. Consumers of this information have come to expect vital healthcare information on how to prevent dreadful infectious diseases resulting in egregiously high death rates. The current Coronavirus (COVID-19) pandemic serves as a convenient example. Time is of the essence in communicating updates about such diseases to members of the public who are anxious to consume information for self-examination and to implement recommendations from international and local health organizations as well as new governmental policies as they are made available. The question is, are journalists keeping up with the demand for health information?

The emergence of online publications was proceeded by the right granted to sell media content on the internet by Nigerian Communications Commission (NCC) in 1996. It licensed 38 internet service providers granting them permission to serve the Nigerian market. In 2000, the internet began to expand. It was below one percent of the Nigerian market then and over the next seven years rose to seven percent.[10] This indicates that officially, the right to practice print media journalism on the internet as a government approved licensed publishing establishment represents a positive move for new print digital media organizations and freelancers. This has given rise to private publications and ordinary people participating in journalism.

The internet was already redefining the practice of journalism when the NCC began licensing service providers in 1996. This provided a boost to the presence and entrepreneurship of Nigerian print media. At this point in time, digital utilization of such an awesome opportunity for the easy distribution of essential healthcare information to Nigerian citizens should not be an issue but it is.

For instance, the digital print media *Sahara Reporters* founded by Nigerian politician Omoyele Sowore. As an ambitious political activist, Sowore focuses his content on politics. Those active in the healthcare arena might learn from this example and be encouraged to promote healthcare content.

The problem is that only a limited number of entrepreneurs are focusing on healthcare. No one blames a journalist whose interest is in politics rather than healthcare or medical information. But this is the root cause of the content imbalance on healthcare. At least some journalists need to focus on healthcare content. Publications devoted to healthcare are needed. Healthcare issues need a constant presence in the media.

The number of print digital media in Nigeria is on the rise. Some digital content publishers in Nigeria include WORDKRAFT Communications Limited, Nigerian OrientNews, Zedek Resources Publishing Ministry, ICIDR Publishing House, Ikot-Ekpene, 1st October Publication Limited, publications from Hoofbeat.com Nigeria Publishers, and *PAROUSIA Magazine*.[11] As a result, news accessibility has been made easy by the availability of these and other new publishing companies functioning in different locations throughout the country. This has resulted in a tremendous advancement in the technical means for the dissemination of news.

The presence of print media on digital platforms transformed the industry and promotes the versatility of its reach to readers. Publishing firms are largely depending on digital print media in making impacts in their various communities and Nigeria. Lives are being transformed through this process and readers seem to crave more content.

Initially, it was viewed that print media was being disrupted but through the technology advancement in virtual digital; it was but not in the manner initially thought. The industry was being saved. Digital print media provides more agents of transformation and quickly serves the ongoing need for new and relevant information of readers. This is reflected in the feedback and posts of readers' comments on digital print media. People feel more well educated when consuming news.

Factors Responsible for Content Imbalance

ADVERTISING DEGRADES DELIVERY OF HEALTHCARE CONTENT

Every business requires funds to maintain operations. The print media, in most cases, are motivated by the desire to fund their operations through commercials. They willingly divert readers' attention from content to commercial advertisements in a quest to retaining sponsors and the associated flow of revenue. Readers who are fed with commercial content featuring products and services are distracted from consuming healthcare or other socially valuable information. This diminishes the benefit the public could otherwise derive from timely and useful healthcare information necessary for a healthy society which becomes part of the background noise in the media.

"Advertising is any paid form of communication from an identified sponsor or source that draws attention to ideas, goods, services or the sponsor itself. Most advertising is directed towards groups rather than individuals, and advertising is usually delivered through media."[12] Most readers see the media as an institution that is losing a connection to its essential function with the focus on too much advertising. This distracts from the media serving its primary function of informing, educating, enlightening, and sharing socially valuable information including healthcare messages.

As stated in an abstract of a case study written by Ahmed Tanimu Jibril of Bauchi State University, Gadau, Nigeria, "the multimodal nature of the present-day advertisements has accorded the genre some tremendous unseen power, capable of influencing people's choices, when it comes to accepting ideas or goods and services."[13] Jibril asserts that commercial advertisements are necessary but that they ought to align with the media objectives as a dimensional tool for the media to use in covering healthcare and other socially valuable issues. Obviously, media organizations need sources of funding and running commercial advertisements serves that function. The issue is the excessive flood of commercials leads to neglect of the healthcare sector, thereby, preventing the media from taking a proactive stance in preventing or mitigating the impact of infectious diseases.

Too much advertising focused only on products and services appear in newspapers, magazines, bulletins, and other print publications. This degrades the quality of service expected of print media in reaching out to the public on healthcare issues of interest to the public. For instance, the COVID-19 pandemic should not have come as a surprise to the Nigerian people. The print media had enough time to reach out to those in the rural areas before COVID-19 hit Nigeria but they were sluggish in sharing information about it or paid little attention as though it was a disease that had only foreign impact. Unfortunately, it turned out to be a global pandemic as announced by World Health Organization (WHO) on March 11, 2020.

There are numerous advertisements saturating Nigerian media today. Some of these advertisements have no healthcare information infused in them. No matter the product or services being advertised in a commercial, most ads could contain some recommendation of beneficial healthcare behavior in conformance with information or cautions provided by international and local healthcare organizations but there are some associated challenges with this approach.

Unfortunately, "the more you read, the less you benefit" is becoming the norm in the media. Undeniably, most advertisements only occupy space without gaining readers' attention. Readers are quick to turn printed pages of publications and the same applies to scrolling through digital print online publications. Studies have proven that print ads are predominantly being ignored by readers. "The top reason consumers said they ignore print ads is because they see print ads too frequently."[14]

Medical companies are helping fill the gap on the provision of healthcare information to the public at a time when serious medical information is needed in the society. They are professional scientific medical officials which is good but they are not actually journalists.

"Like every other field, there are ethical issues in health communication because the media faces the dilemma of making choices daily. Journalists who communicate health information should not compromise ethical principles for commercial gains or purposes."[15] This is a critical issue in health communication. Healthcare information communicated via commercials serves two purposes. It promotes the product and it instructs on necessary healthcare requirements and policies. Private medical organizations may sponsor publications, programs, and articles while also communicating an awareness of the relevant diseases while at the same time advertising their products and services. The issue with disseminating public health information in this manner is that it can demote the impact of the information on the readers and sometimes creates confusion in the mind of the reader.

The advertisements presented by medical companies on print media are generally very creative and stylish to compete with counterparts and grab the attention of consumers. When advertisements are seen as a source for informing readers on a dangerous disease, the how the information is perceived by the consumer can be divided. It all depends on which of the messages the reader chooses to digest, is it the product in question or the underlying awareness on the disease that the advertisement conveys? This can cause confusion because these advertisements appear in various forms. Some provide comic relief by demonstrating something that might have gone wrong, swaying the readers to laughter. This can distract entirely from a primary healthcare issue and completely lose the essence of the message. The ad might offer a cartoon displaying comedic characters involved in a serious situation, thus losing the effectiveness and impact of the healthcare information.

Why do you ignore print advertising in magazines and newspapers from companies?	Satisfied Customers	Unsatisfied Customers
I see print ads too frequently	19%	21%
Their print ads are not relevant to me	15%	22%
The print ads are not interesting	14%	22%
I don't have time to read them	17%	18%
They can't hold my attention	15%	19%
Print ads are too focused on the companies' needs, and not enough on my needs	10%	14%
Don't trust print ads to provide me the information I need to make purchase decisions	8%	13%
Print ads seem like they serve other people's needs, not people like me	9%	11%
Other reasons	2%	4%

The above data on print advertising was generated by MarektingSherpa in a survey of 2400 consumers.[16]

The bottom line is that advertisements represent a huge distraction for readers who depend on print media for news on healthcare in Nigeria. Obviously, media businesses depend on advertising to generate the revenues they need to operate but this creates a conflict of interest situation where the activities of advertising are distracting from the primary service of the media organization in serving the public interest for socially useful and beneficial information.

Covering all aspects of communication from every necessary angle to keep the public abreast on the happenings around them and their environment is what places all media channels above other sectors. For instance, in the case of COVID-19, the delay in providing timely information to the public contributed to the penetration of this deadly disease in Nigeria. The media was saturated with ads but slow to provide proactive communications on border closures for travelers and preparations for isolation centers with medical equipment like ventilators, drugs, kits, test tools, and more. The COVID-19 situation was not managed in an expeditious and effective manner. This was indicated by the absence of valuable healthcare information. Nigerian print media could have championed COVID-19 announcements and updates from when it first surfaced in the world. This might have drawn more government and public attention toward the need to preemptively act. Rather the issue was noticed in print publications only after some officials who traveled for meetings were identified as positive for COVID-19.

The first case of Coronavirus was confirmed in Lagos on February 27, 2020. "The Federal Ministry of Health has confirmed a coronavirus disease (COVID-19) case in Lagos State, Nigeria. The case, which was confirmed on the 27th of February 2020, is the first case to be reported in Nigeria since the beginning of the outbreak in China in January 2020."[17] This was a wake-up call, though it came too late to stop the disease from spreading throughout the country. The print media was expected to take such issues seriously by reporting on how other countries or regions affected were handling the pandemic and what Nigerians could do to protect themselves against this disease but they failed to do so in an effective manner.

ENTERTAINMENT MORE POPULAR THAN HEALTHCARE INFORMATION

Nigerian print media places too much value on entertainment news in comparison to healthcare content addressing infectious diseases in news publications as a basis for their business operations. "It is both an exciting and challenging time for the media and entertainment sector. As online and social media become more popular, traditional outlets are having to reassess a business model that has served them well for many years. This is happening at a time when macroeconomic factors are dampening demand for services and sponsorship, while also increasing costs."[18] This observation highlights the increased reshaping of the Nigerian media industry in regard to sponsorship and finance that favors entertainment news.

As an example, Nigerian print media recently promoted entertainment stories about Nollywood stars and their families in an effort to maintain their relevance in the minds of the fans and the general public. Many famous actors, actresses, musicians, comedians, and artists of all sorts are becoming a daily conversation that distracts readers who seek healthcare information in print media. Given the traditional role of print media in serving the public interest, it is alarming that so much importance is attached to fame promotion of people whose faces appear on television entertainment programs. The market place is filled with papers and magazines showing photos of the so-called star faces and articles spreading gossip of their activities in abandonment of health facts and information associated with diseases currently ravaging the world.

Examples of Nigerian entertainment magazines on print papers and print digital media include *Bella Naija, Buzz Nigeria, Nija Gists, Ovation Magazine, Yaba Left, Happenings Magazine, TW Magazine*, and *Supple Magazine*.[19] These magazines and online publications primarily promote entertainment news and dominate most media content with fictional stories in their quest to gain popularity, funding, and the attention of young readers.

It is difficult if not impossible to find magazines, papers or online publishers devoted entirely to healthcare in Nigeria. Few, if any, healthcare magazines or papers are sold in street venues and those that have attempted this route for distribution often go out of business because they do not stand the taste of public interest and lose financial sponsorships. The stakeholders control production affairs on media with the basic intention of making money or manipulating the subject of public interest via Nigeria media. The focus in such media on star power makes one wonder if healthcare is not as relevant as fictional actors. Yet, a huge amount of money is still spent in support of medical and science students compared to those studying the Arts. The question is, are medical and healthcare practitioners not worthy of high recognition like these famous Nollywood stars? Are Nigerian scientists not making impacts in the society to the same or a greater extent than the famous Nigerian actors, actresses, and artists?

This could be as a result of the high number of youths in the general population compared to elderly people. Young people tend to care less about health issues favoring the excitement and glamour of show business. Which arena has more pull on Nigerian youths deciding upon a career? The irony is that medical workers and scientists are viewed as unemployed or underpaid, while popular entertainers are being projected in print media as wealthy achievers. This is the result of journalists and the publishing companies allowing society control the content and narrative that is presented for public consumption. This self-fulfilling trend has eaten deep in the system, exemplified by the fact that the active generation cares less about healthcare compared to entertainment.

Journalists who further this trend seem to have forgotten the responsibilities of their traditional role, believing they succeed by having readers who patronize them and revenue generated from the interviews they gather on Nollywood stars and artists seeking fame and fortune themselves. Meanwhile, the responsibility to serve the interests of humanity is forgotten.

Consider the relationship between a mother and her baby. How should a mother decide what to feed her baby? Should she choose only what the baby demands or what is good nutritional food that will allow the baby to develop as a healthy human being? There is little difference in what the print media feeds the public. When the media is saturated with entertainment content rather than maintaining at least a balance with healthcare information, the resulting decline in public health should be expected.

Regulations for balancing content creation have been downplayed in the media and by some public figures. For the most part, society is no longer encouraged to keep researching and scientifically proving facts, rather many individuals consume entertainment news with the aspiration of becoming a star someday, somehow. That is the general perspective presented by the print media.

Entertainers are seen as the role models to a greater extent than healthcare officials whose lives are on the line every day in an effort to save humanity from various ailments and diseases. Fighting COVID-19 in an environment like Nigeria with the entertainment industry ruling print media content is certainly a wake-up call. But is it being heeded? It does, however, remind journalists of the gap they have accepted and created as promoters of entertainment with a corresponding decline in attention to healthcare issues.

RELIGION DIVERTS ATTENTION FROM VALID HEALTHCARE ISSUES

Religion offers another dimension of journalism that floods the print media in Nigeria with content. There are uncountable religious publications with little or no healthcare information contained within them. Churches and mosques occupy all corners of the nation and publish newspapers and magazines to promote their own religious interests. Healthcare contents only gain access to the religious publications as articles or warnings when an infectious disease is in active circulation. These magazines do not have regular pages for the promotion of healthy practices.

Religious institutions are expected through their publications to encourage health workers, health organizations, governmental efforts, and any health-related administration in the pursuit of saving the human race from dangerous diseases and infections through the dissemination of relevant medical warnings as regular content of their publications. This is part of the life-saving efforts expected to keep filling the need for health maintenance contents in Nigerian paper and ICT print media.

"Beyond their legal and ethical relationship, in the context of politics, religion and media intimately connect in a number of ways. The media serve as communicating instrument for religion. Religion uses the media as vehicles for religious propagation and proselytization. In addition to patronising the media owned by others, many religious organisations with the wherewithal, today, own various types of media outlets."[20] The fact is that the influence of media on religion is undeniable and the need to function for mass communication which is essential to the progress of modern church and the society. Religion is expected to provide a certain level of health content coverage in service of its role in Corporate Social Responsibility (CSR) to the Nigerian people.

SUPERNATURAL INFORMATION PERVADES MEDIA

Nigerian society has been saturated with stories of miraculous healing in print media. This prompts church members to seek healthcare remedies from their pastors instead of medical professionals, believing that healing is a matter of faith alone. This resulted in church members developing a high dependency on pastors rather than doctors until the recent pandemic proved the fallacy of this approach. Pastors, of course, were not able to heal individuals infected with COVID-19. Church officials certainly do not want to risk contracting the Corona virus in the process of trying to heal a church member. If pastors could reverse the impact of the virus, the rich and famous members of the community infected with COVID-19 would have flocked to the churches but that didn't happen. "Life-threatening illness can bring anyone face to face with the supernatural."[21] However, reality is often a harsh arbitrator of the truth. Nearly everyone in communities throughout Nigeria now seek help from medical professionals in an effort to survive the COVID-19 global pandemic. Hospitals and health centers have suddenly become very popular. While religious people do pray for God to provide a cure for COVID-19, it is asked that it be delivered through medical scientists, doctors, and other medical professionals, not the church.

Print media to a large degree has also been overtaken by supernatural beliefs and speculations on the existence of miraculous cures with make-belief and fake practices gaining public attention and followership while consumers of this disinformation willingly disregard reality and scientific norms on how the healing process actually works. The recent pandemic has proven that misleading individuals for profit or personal gain works until one is revealed in the light of the reality of the situation. Healthcare is about reality. Learning the medical principles of dealing with deadly infectious diseases by experience is a risky path for anyone, especially when dealing with COVID-19 or Ebola that have proven to be speedy killers.

Obviously, Coronavirus is not an infection with which to play. It demands urgent medical attention and has highlighted the importance of adhering to health protocols in a manner learned from Ebola in 2014. The fear of COVID-19 pandemic penetrated the entirety of Nigeria and garnered public attention when people known to the public were being infected and dying. This was not about the wealthy or poor. COVID-19 carries the risk of death for anyone seriously infected. Couple that with the fact that a cure is not yet available. The seriousness of this threat has prompted the closure of many international borders making the mantra, "save yourself in your own country" even more important. The Coronavirus serves as a serious public lesson on the importance of professional healthcare and medical attention on an individual basis and for those occupying a particular space or community.

OVERUSE OF PUBLIC ALERTS DIMINISHES ATTENTION TO HEALTHCARE ISSUES

Print news is the cornerstone of media information distribution for Nigerian readers but it is becoming less important in terms of actual news since newspapers have diminished the amount of healthcare content. Additionally, *BREAKING NEWS!* alerts have begun to replace in depth news coverage on a variety of issues. These alerts have become so common that they are beginning to be seen as a cliché in the print media industry. Their use is a bid to gain readers' attention but usually, when the attention of the reader is successfully gained, it turns out that the information is not important enough to deserve the time wasted in reading it. In actuality, healthcare information should occupy most of the space reserved for serious alerts but they are not used until the death toll in victims have become unbearably high.

Readers' attention can be drawn to facts and reality in the healthcare section and interest amplified when readers turn the page and see *ANNOUNCEMENT!* The information gains popularity, impact and becomes more effective but the page must contain information that is useful to the reader. Readers hunger and thirst for healthcare news but, recently, the media has made little or no space available on a regular basis for healthcare news alerts.

Serious readers complain of little or no healthcare information on the important pages and deceitful headlines that divert their attention from the important health information they seek. Healthcare campaigns, medical treatments for infections, available cures for diseases, health policies, health warnings from organizations on health cases, new health habits and other vital information is expected from the alerts in print media but instead, readers are distracted while the media shoves irrelevant content in readers' faces. This results in important healthcare programs or events taking place without adequate public notification by the print media. Journalists have the obligation of providing the public timely healthcare reports and alerts especially when important public officials are involved in an event. Even international healthcare programs that should not be disregarded, sometimes do not receive adequate public notification in the print media.

Alerting readers on healthcare events requires a professional approach to provide the public with information that is consistent and timely fulfilling the goal of proper notification. One-time publication of alerts about the event may not suffice. Print media must partner with producers of the event to create successful notification of the public. Some healthcare programs lack attendance because the public were not alerted at the right time with accurate information about the events and their importance to public health.

Reports on medical achievements provide good information but, in many cases, are too often ignored even when heroes in the medical field emerge from them. Healthcare officials, nurses, medical doctors and other healthcare professionals who sacrifice their personal time and lives in the interest of public health are not usually highlighted in the alert sections of the print media. Their duty and achievements are often more important in terms of public health than alerts that are currently published with the headline *ATTENTION! BREAKING NEWS! NEWS ALERT!*

POLITICS PREEMPTS IMPORTANT HEALTHCARE INFORMATION

Since the inception of media in Nigeria, political content has always been highlighted in the headlines. This might be expected since many of Nigerian newspapers were founded to serve political interests and mainly serve to promote regional and national political interests. Politics in print media has always overlapped other content, pointing to the origin of print media in Nigeria that traces back to the political struggle by prominent figures involved in Nigerian Independence. Such political partisanship has always been the major component of Nigerian print media since the period preceding independence. It all began with the emergence of *West African Pilot*, the first Nigerian-owned English language newspaper founded in 1937 by the first Nigerian President Nnamdi Azikiwe. The *West African Pilot* served strictly to support the independence struggle during the colonial era. Also catering to state or regional interests are the *Eastern Nigerian Guardian*, launched in Port Harcourt; *The Southern Defender* in Warri; *The Sentinel* in Enugu; and the *Northern Advocate* in Jos. Azikiwe's newspaper defended the Eastern Region agenda. Obafemi Awolowo launched the Nigerian Tribune in 1949 in Ibadan five years before he became the premier of the Western Region and advocated for the interests of that region. Nigerian political history is embedded in today's media and produces a continuing imbalance in terms of content presented to readers.

The leadership struggle and power intoxication has been the bone of contention in streamlining Nigeria media almost as a complete political arena neglecting other sectors as minor discussion in papers. Another leading daily read newspaper, *The Sun* was founded by Orji Uzor Kalu in 2001. This was two years after his successful election as the governor of Abia State. Kalu also launched a sister daily publication called the *New Telegraph*. The trend of newspapers based on politics keeps emerging as *The Nation*, one of the top newspapers, was founded in 2006 by Bola Ahmed Tinubu, then an opposition politician who aided in the formation of the All Progressive Congress (APC) in an effort to compete against the strength of the People's Democratic Party (PDP) that later succeeded in winning the 2015 and 2019 elections in Nigeria. These achievements accomplished through the use of print media by the political interests which dominates them still influences Nigerian media today.[22]

The role of the print media in Nigeria nearly always defers to political interests resulting in the diminution of the proper responsibility and role of the media and journalists in serving the public interest. This leaves citizens with little or no choice regarding the content they receive. Healthcare is easily subjugated to content that serves political interests in newspapers throughout Nigeria.

Recommendations

These recommendations serve as processes to be recognized in correcting issues in connection to contributing factors responsible for content imbalance.

USE OF ADVERTISEMENTS TO ADDRESS HEALTHCARE

Most media advertisements serve as a vehicle for fast penetration in the society regarding specific products and services. Introducing creative but valid healthcare content as part of their delivery can help educate the public on these issues. This can aid in the improvement of readers' behavior when it comes to healthy lifestyles. The more readers see such content on different advertisements, the more it will influence their habits and behaviors. Ultimately, this will help improve public health.

BALANCING OF HEALTHCARE CONTENT ADVISED

Print media in Nigeria needs government regulation to guide the inclusion of healthcare information in its regular content. There is need for improvements in the structural mandates for publication of news on diseases and infections. More medical news, health and scientific contents, health campaigns and programs updates, health policies by government, health information from organizations and healthcare officials of both international and local affairs are needed to create a better balance in the media content availability for readers. It is an obligation of the print media to provide the society with reliable reports from credible sources on healthy living for an active society. The issue of providing content based on popular demand or interest rigging should not affect the availability of health content that benefits society.

HEALTHCARE INFORMATION PROMOTION ON PRINT ICT MEDIA AND PAPER PRINT MEDIA

Increased utilization of print ICT-based media to attract the new generation to healthcare content is advisable. Heroes of healthcare need to be celebrated as global and national heroes. Attention to these champions will raise recognition of their accomplishments in Nigeria and elsewhere on the internet and in other media. The high population of digital media users who focus on personal media chats could potentially be redirected to matters of more social urgency including the life-saving reality of health information. The greater availability of content on healthcare could provide such an audience with the information they need to avoid falling victim to infections and diseases. Digital print media offers a fast reach to nearly any location throughout the country for the distribution of healthcare information. Influencing the new generation on healthcare deals could make a significant difference in how quickly infectious disease are able to spread throughout the country.

CONSISTENCY

Print media publications need to consistently feature information about diseases, medicals and scientific discoveries, healthcare policies, guidance from healthcare workers, and warnings or advisories. Typically, once an outbreak is declared over, the print media reduces and sometimes abandons completely the publication of important healthcare information. Journalists should be attentive to the fact that it is necessary to keep updating the public consistently on these topics by referencing healthcare campaigns, events, and tragic effects of an outbreak in order to help to prevent future outbreaks of the disease or emergence of new infections. Journalists should uphold their social responsibilities by providing the essential healthcare information to the public on a regular basis.

SALARY OF HEALTHCARE JOURNALISTS

The issue of how much healthcare journalists are paid relates to the problem of lack of healthcare content in the media. Low pay for journalists creates the incentive for other sectors of society, especially politics and entertainment, to leverage undue influence in regard to the content that appears in the print media. Operational funding and journalists' salary levels reside at the root of the temptation to preempt important healthcare information with other content. It also contributes to the lack of dedicated healthcare journalists. Healthy journalists covering healthcare issues sends a positive message to the public about the benefit of living a healthy lifestyle. Journalists are better able to attend to self-care and maintenance when they earn a good salary for their work. It will also demonstrate the benefits of their career choice and attract new journalists to the industry. Unfortunately, a memo from Punch management to its staff reflects the reality of what journalists must endure especially during the COVID-19 pandemic lockdown. "Considering the fact on the ground and the body movement of the board, full salaries may not be paid in May and some people, especially in the newsroom, would be forced to resign."[23] This issue demands an urgent solution to save the healthcare sector in Nigerian print journalism from experiencing a self-perpetuating spiral of decline.

MORE HEALTHCARE PRINT MEDIA COMPANIES, JOURNALISTS, SCIENCE, AND MEDICALS REQUIRED

The healthcare sector in Nigeria needs a serious infusion of support from the government, organizations, institutions, and the private sector. The health of Nigerian society depends upon quick action. There is need for more newspapers, magazines, journals, books, and digital publications from existing and emerging print media companies to focus solely on healthcare. There is an urgent need in this area. The availability of more publishing companies focused on healthcare content will help prove the relevance of healthcare information to members of Nigeria society. It will facilitate the distribution of life-saving healthcare information to the public which will contribute to a positive transformation in the general health of the public in the country.

PROFESSIONAL JOURNALISTS ON HEALTHCARE SURVEILLANCE

The fact is that healthcare journalists who are persistent and work hard to ensure that healthcare content is balanced with other issues in print publications do exist. It takes those who are called to do their jobs with passion and care for humanity to fulfill this great role. These devoted journalists are the movers of public healthcare communication via print media in Nigeria. They are helping to rectify the imbalance of healthcare content. They provide information on healthy habits and cautions regarding the novel COVID-19 pandemic. Many of these journalists work for healthcare newspapers, magazines or journals, and digital print publications that represent private firms that are focused on regularly updating their readers on COVID-19 information.

They report the number of individuals infected and death rates, while informing the public on the dangers of not adhering to health warnings and new compliance orders. Healthcare headlines, such as "Deaths in Nigerian city raise concerns over undetected Covid-19 outbreaks," as well as "Coronavirus – latest updates" and "See all our coronavirus coverage"[24] offer good examples of information published in online newspapers in an effort to keep the public abreast on COVID-19 issues. The print media journalists who work for these outlets coordinate with the Nigeria Centre for Disease Control (NCDC) on latest newsworthy updates in relation to COVID-19 and other healthcare issues. NCDC also communicates COVID-19 cases directly to the public through its digital online publications.

As an example, NCDC COVID-19 reports on the infection and its spread as of August 16, 2020, indicated:[25]

- Total Number of Cases – 49,068
- Total Number Discharged – 36,497
- Total Deaths – 975
- Total Tests Carried out – 350,589

According to the NCDC, "298 new cases were reported from 16 Nigerian states as follows: Plateau (108), Kaduna (49), Lagos (47), Ogun (18), Osun (17), FCT (15), Ondo (14), Edo (8), Oyo (6), Akwa Ibom (4), Cross River (4), Borno (3), Ekiti (2), Bauchi (1), Kano (1), and Rivers (1)."

"Meanwhile, the latest numbers bring Lagos state total confirmed cases to 16,503, followed by Abuja (4,729), Oyo (2,958), Edo (2,431), Rivers (2,006), Plateau (1,816), Kaduna (1,815), Kano (1,679), Delta (1,639), Ogun (1,563), Ondo (1,395), Enugu (997), Ebonyi (931), Kwara (906), Osun (754), Katsina (746), Borno (706), Abia (677), Gombe (676), and Bauchi (583). Imo State has recorded 506 cases, Benue (430), Nasarawa (374), Bayelsa (352), Jigawa (322), Akwa Ibom (250), Niger (229), Ekiti (206), Adamawa (185), Anambra (156), Sokoto (154), Kebbi (90), Taraba (78), Zamfara and Cross River (77), and Yobe (67) while Kogi has recorded five cases only."

These results above are reported by professionals who perform their journalistic duties while risking their lives sourcing news amidst COVID-19 outbreaks in various communities throughout Nigeria. They deserve commendation and encouragement to continue their good work.

CITIZEN JOURNALISM ON PRINT DIGITAL MEDIA IMPROVING HEALTHCARE

Augmenting the volume of healthcare news content provided to the public, citizen journalism emerges on the internet from anywhere, at any time, and by anyone as a viable option to fill the gap. These new entrepreneurs in the healthcare journalism seem passionate about the communication of public healthcare information. Some are medical practitioners while others emerge as healthcare publishers through training, education or other experience in the medical field. This new career path provides job opportunities while at the same time improving the wellbeing of Nigerian society.

The issue with this new development is, traditional print media managers, who gate-keep content before release or publication have no control over these independent or private online publishers. There are at least two billion internet users in the world making cyber space a popular public arena for the exchange of information. This does not make healthcare web bloggers professional journalists. There are rules in journalism that ordinary participants may not know about or abide by because they lack media training on them. This is why they are not legally allowed to claim their roles as journalists.

Some healthcare online magazines are owned by medical doctors or health workers who take up the obligations of media practitioners in an effort to confront health matters on the internet. "A number of Nigerian entrepreneurs are entering the printing business [...] although there is no local manufacture of printing and graphic arts equipment, most major publications use fairly sophisticated machines."[26]

"In the past decade, new communication technologies, particularly network communication, have made it possible for others also to publish content for a potentially global audience. Of course, the arena of public communication and especially healthcare news reliability is still championed by healthcare print media journalists as a proven content, although citizen journalism on digital media, undeniably poses a challenge to print media journalists. Thus, institutional journalism has encountered for the first time a serious challenge to its social function, an activity parallel to its own."[27]

Some of these online healthcare publishers provide aid for healthcare professional journalists by being the first-hand news informants on healthcare issues online, while the journalists verify, report, edit, and print or publish the information online in a professional and proper way. Gate-keeping achieved by traditional print media through the processes involved in newsroom produces accurate content worthy of being trusted by consumers of the information. This distinguishes the citizen journalism from professional media journalism.

The public benefit which distinguishes print news media from online free journalism businesses "establishes a strong case for requiring platforms to give advance warning of changes which significantly affect news media business operations and revenues. In more general terms, it is reasonable to regard digital platforms as having a duty not to harm the public benefit provided by news and journalistic content."[28]

PARTNERSHIPS BETWEEN JOURNALISTS AND HEALTHCARE PROFESSIONALS IN TRAINING JOURNALISTS

Partnerships between medical media journalists and medical professionals who produce healthcare content helps provide the public with timely and accurate medical updates, news on healthy living, and health maintenance information. The information might not reach the public as anticipated because of financial support and sponsorship but this is still a useful partnership. People depend on publications and publications have readers distributed throughout the nation. This is one of the reasons why the Federal

Ministry of Health in partnership with the WHO have organized workshop training for journalists and editors covering health activities in Nigeria (Abuja) in an effort to achieve basic public healthcare objectives. These training sessions help ensure the mobilization of professional journalists to counter any negative reporting regarding public health intervention programs. This improves the knowledge and skill of journalists in reporting, writing, and editing stories about disease outbreaks and other healthcare issues.[29]

These workshops also provide journalists with first-hand information from key program officers on the support provided by the WHO to the government of Nigeria. It empowers journalists with knowledge on how best to write and edit healthcare stories. Such training encourages journalists on the need to investigate and ensure data-based and evidence-based health reporting while orienting journalists on the communication framework and community engagement models employed by the WHO. The Hon. Minister of Health, Prof. Isaac Adewole, represented by the Director of Media and Public Relations for the Federal Ministry of Health (FMOH), Mrs. Boade Akinola, said that health issues are not a one-man business. "It is a collective responsibility of all stakeholders including media practitioners." This was quoted from a speech delivered at one of the trainings held in Nigeria. It also justifies and encourages the valuable partnership between professional journalists and healthcare professionals in the dissemination of important health information to the public.

TRAINING AND AWARDING OF JOURNALISTS FOR HEALTHCARE COVERAGE

The Hon. Minister of Health, Prof. Isaac Adewole "said that health journalists had great role to play in providing the public with information aimed at preventing and controlling disease outbreaks in Nigeria. He urged the trained journalists to bring to bear, the knowledge acquired during the training in the practice of their profession. He added that Ministry of Health and the WHO office were planning to initiate a journalists Award to those who perform excellently in their reportage."[30] In support of this assertion, the WHO communication specialist, Ms. Charity Warigon urged journalists to work hard and focus more on investigative reporting. She said, "reward for hard work is certain, though it may not come immediately, but it would eventually come." She discouraged the use of sensationalism in reporting on healthcare issues in Nigeria because it distorts facts and has the potential for causing havoc.

As the report points out, the participants of the WHO training were drawn from print, electronic and online media. It is expected that the award to journalists will boost the desire of journalists to engage in professional media practices in regard to healthcare content disseminated by Nigerian media industry. This is a commendable initiative by the Nigerian Ministry of Health and the WHO.

PRINT ICT-BASED MEDIA ON HEALTHCARE

Publishers are constantly trying to reframe the operational models for healthcare digital news on the internet to engage the young generation. "Social Media has played a major impact on how we receive our daily news. Many people decide to get the news from apps on their phones, because it is convenient to read."[31] This makes it easier for consumers of the news to discuss and provide feedback. As a result, numerous versions of online publications have emerged. Currently, digital news from print media has garnered the attention of Nigerian journalists. The amount of information now obtainable from digital communications was unimaginable only decades earlier. The world is globally informed today like never before and the ease of access to healthcare news provides readers who seek health content with hope for better balance in the content they receive.

"Communication in human society has come a very long way. From the primitive era, through the era of supremacy of the mainstream media to the emerging era of reign of the new media, communication has remained the live wire of the society. Odii (2013, p.160), observed that the apparatus and styles of communication keep changing. This generational dynamism in communication tools and systems has resulted in astounding evolution of a collaborative, participatory, democratic and user-generated- content pattern of communication. Massive technological changes over the past decade have created new opportunities for freedom of expression and information."[32]

Print digital content publishers on healthcare are also changing the game in terms of their content delivery via the internet. They are reformists, redefining the pattern of how consumers engage with content online, by focusing more on the quality of audience engagement than the quantity of participants. Consider the fact that authors' identities are now presented with their posts online making it easier to direct feedback to the provider.

"Technological development has led the media to both expand and retract. Digital transmission has resulted in more and cheaper opportunities for broadcasters and greater choice for media consumers."[33]

The fact that consumers can easily access healthcare news via traditional print media as well as with the new digital devices facilitates the distribution of information that contributes to the provision of general healthcare to society. More people participating in the process of sharing information as bloggers, commentators, and writers on the internet as *citizen journalists* as distinguished from professional journalists expands the amount of health information reaching the public. And, given the ease for consumers to provide feedback on the quality and benefit of the information they receive, all the mechanisms are in place for an effective distribution and feedback loop that only help to improve the level of content provided.

CHAPTER TWO

Influence of Media Campaign on Positive Healthcare Behavioral Change and Social Transformation

Overview

Traces of good evidence exist that public health communication in Nigeria has had an effect on the wellbeing of the society. As seen in Julie Leask et al, *Media Coverage of Health Issues and How to Work More Effectively with Journalists: A Qualitative Study*, "Public health professionals have always been sensitive to the persuasive power of the mass media. In fact, public health has often had the challenging task of both using the media to influence health practices while countering this same influence where it encourages unhealthy choices."[1]

Trends indicate that public health communication or education and health behavior of individuals have yielded very positive results. A huge change is discovered in the health behavior of individuals traced in many spheres of lifestyles and habitual activities as the media keeps communicating the dangers implications if the public does not adhere to the directives of healthcare officials. Consider the following health issues: smoking, blood pressure control, cholesterol consumption, condom use, high sugar consumption, stress management, nutrition, and social distancing, etc. Health awareness campaigns in these areas have proven effective, with positive feedback detected from the behavioral change of the populace as determined by the healthcare services of Nigeria.

Some healthcare issues related to behavioral changes are monitored in public communication and relate to a particular habit of the public that if changed could aid in the prevention of diseases and ailments through the educational efforts of the media. Some of these activities or programs include the National High Blood Pressure Education Program, anti-smoking campaigns, sudden infant death syndrome education, AIDS Communication Program, highway safety programs, antidrug medical campaigns, and efforts by the Nigeria Center for Disease Control (NCDC) that was established by law in November, 2018. The NCDC is also concerned with managing the COVID-19 outbreak in Nigeria which has blossomed into a global pandemic ravaging the world. These are some of the public healthcare communication programs and platforms that have contributed immensely to healthcare improvement and disease prevention in Nigeria.

"Mass media campaigns can work through direct and indirect pathways to change the behavior of whole populations. Many campaigns aim to directly affect individual recipients by invoking cognitive or emotional responses. Such programs are intended to affect decision-making processes at the individual level. Anticipated outcomes include the removal or lowering of obstacles to change, helping people to adopt healthy or recognize unhealthy social norms, and to associate valued emotions with achieving change."[2] These campaigns can take the form of direct and indirect approaches to behavioral change.

The direct pathway to behavioral change is when new behaviors are achieved through media campaigns. Hygiene is one of the most effective campaign topics for improving public behaviors during an infection outbreak. It produces some of the highest returns for the investment at both the national and global levels. A simple example is washing hands with soap which is also one of the most cost-effective health interventions. Unfortunately, hygiene is too often neglected in aftermath of an infection crises.[3]

The outbreak of a disease raises alarms and often invokes fear which can cause behavioral change. The direct threat of infections or disease detections can be an effective driver for major immediate social change toward the adoption of new, healthier behaviors. These are achieved through media campaigns as a source of positive influence on public health behaviors and can bring about a social transformation in a particular community. This is evident in "public policy efforts and government campaigns to promote hygiene practices. Handwashing with soap captures a miniscule proportion of national health budgets and international aid spending on health – typically less than 1%. Part of the reason for the lack of funding is the uncertainty around what makes behavior change campaigns a success and the prospect of a return on investments."[4]

When the WHO strongly affirmed a toolkit for healthcare communication designed to curb the spread of infection during the Ebola outbreak in 2014, compliance was achieved completely and every community was closely monitored as a compulsory task. Nigerian media played their role in sensitizing the public on the need for this practice. The public accepted the information and commendable results were realized.

Introduction of the program Communication for Behavioral Impact (COMBI) by the WHO proved to be very successful.[5] Such a public health imperative during an outbreak helps bring the event under control as quickly as possible, minimizing morbidity, mortality, and other negative impacts of dangerous diseases. The impact was realized as people adapted to a new norm. Such efforts are commendable and their continuation is necessary in all spheres of healthcare behavioral change.

The COMBI toolkit offered by the WHO needs to be understood more broadly and applied to guide changes in public behavior, culture, economy, society, and politics when appropriate for effective behavioral change. It reveals potential routes for amplification and transmission embedded in deep-seated cultural practices critical for adapting public behaviors to new normal. The COMBI achieved a specific behavioral result for positive, protective public health results by sensitizing the public on its importance. It also serves as an effective guide for institutions designing response measures to disease outbreaks. It can also be applied at the sub-national and national levels for developmental communication and health promotion in response to disease outbreaks and in guiding behavioral changes. Campaign communication for disease prevention typically demands a huge financial expenditure in order to realize a positive outcome. This has a lot to do with timely outreach to rural areas. This is where the COMBI toolkit serves the essential purpose of providing the prompt delivery of crucial information during an outbreak.

One of the negative strategies that is most effective in invoking fear, which has a negative effect on the public based on social norm, is the use of social media. Social media is useful but can also be harmful in shaping behavior. There might be cases where the information provided by social media misguides the public or conveys a misconception of the information. Given the speed at which information can spread and potentially cause harm among people in a community or globally extreme care must be taken when using social media channels for healthcare campaigns. Nevertheless, lines of support are provided in cases where serious harm might occur. The risks versus benefits might outweigh the potential problems of campaigns using social media to raise the alarm on the dangers for those pursuing or not pursuing particular behaviors.

"Mass media interventions that seek to influence people directly—by directly targeting the people burdened by the public health problem of concern and/or the people who influence them—have a long basis in public health history, and recent reviews have clarified our expectations about what can be expected from such approaches."[6] Most campaign programs generally encourage positive social norms and results-oriented self-regard measures. For instance, an antismoking campaign might emphasize the risks of smoking and the benefits of quitting to boost health and strength while helping to create a more physically active society.

The indirect system of behavioral change is achieved through the interpretation of mass media messages leading to compliance by action. This influences individuals, via interpersonal discussions on health issues within a community's social network or an individual's social group, depending on the intention to undermine particular social behavioral changes.[7] Indirect form of behavioral change among individuals or group influences without the target subjects being exposed to direct campaigns is achieved through indirect infused campaigns. For instance, after reading a newspaper on the risk of smoking, the reader might decide to form or join a group of individuals who have decided to quit smoking. People joining the group may have no direct information from the print media on the behavioral change they seek but they know it is for their own benefit. These members of the group are indirectly influenced resulting in an eventual social transformation.

Such activities transform society in a positive manner through a gradual process. One might not necessarily join a group but still adopt the change of habit as messaged by the group. Also, an individual pursuing the new healthy lifestyle might signal to other people the benefits of living healthy and being free from an addiction. Health campaign behavioral change may directly influence the behavior of various individuals while also indirectly influencing others as a result of the changes made by particular individuals or influencers.

Evidence for large-scale health behavioral change in society is measured by the overall increase or decrease in the percentage of the population complying with the message of direct or indirect campaign set by the media. Maximum effectiveness of any campaign proves its success in a specific individual or as communities demonstrate change to the healthier behavioral norm. This could happen on a regional or national scale and the campaign could target any positive behavior change for a specific set of individuals in a society.

"Mass media interventions that seek to influence people indirectly—by creating beneficial changes in the places (or environments) in which people live and work—have equal if not greater potential to promote beneficial changes in population health behaviors, but these are currently less explored options."[8] It is recommendable for public health program planners to employ media publications and direct campaigns to target people and communities for healthcare behavioral change and compliance in order to obtain the greatest possible benefits. This relies on the fact that the effectiveness of direct approach to community behavioral change is encouraged compared to indirect form of behavioral change especially when speedy outcomes are desired.

An article entitled "Mass Media Campaign Features and Effects on Behaviour" published by the National Center for Biotechnology Information confirmed the existence of strong evidence on the benefit of positive behavioral change as a result of the influence of campaigns on youths addicted to tobacco and other substances.[9] The campaign generally targeted young people and their tobacco consumption, providing information on the negative effects of tobacco on the human body. It sought positive transformation on altering such risky habits among youths.

"Mass media campaigns are widely used to expose high proportions of large populations to messages through routine uses of existing media [...] Exposure to such messages is therefore, generally passive."[10] The print media (magazines, newspapers, journals, and digital ICT) seems to be competitive and market driven aligning with powerful social norms and behaviors.

Media campaigns targeting addictions and habitual transformation have been proven effective over the years. This could involve either be a short or long-term campaign, depending on the expected outcome and goal the campaign is targeted to achieve. A large audience is usually obtained through the media messages during campaigns. Such an approach with print media has shown to be highly effective, particularly with magazines and newspapers. Digital-ICT print media is also championing campaigns involving the new technologies using the internet with mobile phones, computer systems, iPhones, laptops, tablets, and more.

A study of the outcomes of mass media campaigns in the context of most health-risk behaviors concluded "that mass media campaigns can produce positive changes or prevent negative changes in health-related behaviors across large populations." Contributors to these outcomes are "the concurrent availability of required services and products, availability of community-based program, and policies that support behavior change." Suggested areas of improvement include "investment in longer better-funded campaigns to achieve adequate population exposure to media messages."[11]

A successful mass media campaign is obtainable through the media's ability to reach out with definite behavioral focused information to a large target audience or individuals in a community consistently over a long period. This need not come at a high cost. Red alerts that occur sometimes may interrupt this process. Campaign messages do fall short and can incur negative results by not meeting expectations. These could be due to issues not well addressed before embarking on the campaign.

One of significant failure in this area that is still addressed today on Nigerian healthcare campaigns is the Nigerian Health Insurance Scheme (NHIS). Poor government funding of health care and management or oversight of health insurance has hindered the success of NHIS.[12] Informing non-educated Nigerians in the remote villages on healthcare insurance requires meeting with them in person and answering their questions to prove the functionality of the program as designed. This requires sufficient funding by the government for transportation, accommodation, feeding and provision of the necessary tools needed for running the campaign inside villages in order to achieve an effective level of compliance by the rural inhabitants.

Healthcare financial risk protection is still an issue in Nigerian healthcare sector and is the major reason for the failed campaign on Nigerian Health Insurance Scheme (NHIS).[13] The NHIS ought to be well equipped with the campaign requirements to meet up to expectations. The Nigerian government should address this problem to ensure access to quality healthcare services, provide financial risk protection, reduce rising costs of healthcare services, and ensure efficiency in health care. Other healthcare programs requiring funding for a constant campaign to promote healthcare in Nigeria are the National Immunization Coverage Scheme (NICS), Midwives Service Scheme (MSS), Nigerian Pay for Performance Scheme and others. Generally, most unsuccessful media campaigns are the result of inadequate funding.

Social Problems Targeted with Media Campaigns

TOBACCO USE

One of the social problems related to public health behaviors targeted with media campaigns is tobacco use. The target audience mostly involves young people. The success of these campaigns is mostly determined by the availability of resources for changing the type of behavior being addressed. Tobacco use health campaign execution through the media depends largely on its consistency of the content provided until the desired result is achieved. Availability of capital or finance is an essential requirement of a consistent media campaign which must be considered by campaign planners, if not, they have automatically planned to fail from the inception of the program. The tobacco use campaign among youths has not reached out extensively to the populace in rural areas. As a continuous campaign, it ought to be well funded by the government and stakeholders in providing necessary resources needed for a positive outcome.

Ongoing campaigns targeting tobacco use among youths have competing influences with addiction, tobacco marketing, pricing, and social norms.[14] The National Institute of Health (NIH) reviewed the numbers and characteristics of 121 mass media campaigns. It conducted 25 controlled field experiments on youth and 40 on adults along with 57 population-based state/national mass media campaigns (NCI, 2008) and more 11 number of adult-focused with control groups/interrupted time series (Bala et al, 2008). The conclusions drawn from this review process indicate that there is strong evidence demonstrating the benefit the campaigns have on improving the behaviors of the targeted groups.

"Although the agenda for development of a national tobacco control policy dates back to the 1950s, a comprehensive Framework Convention on Tobacco Control (FCTC) compliant policy was only developed in 2015, 10 years after Nigeria signed the FCTC. Lack of funding and conflict of interest (of protecting citizens from harmful effect of tobacco *vis-à-vis* the economic gains from the industry) are the major barriers that slowed the policy process.

The tobacco control effort is fundamentally handicapped by inadequate funding as one of the primary constraints. This needs to change for there to be confidence that such campaigns will produce positive outcomes. "Nigeria has a comprehensive national policy for tobacco control which was formulated a decade after ratification of the FCTC due to constraints of funding and conflict of interest. Not all the tobacco control policies in Nigeria engrain the principles of multisectoral and best buy strategies in their formulation. There is an urgent need to address these neglected areas that may hamper tobacco control efforts in Nigeria."[15]

"Sufficient exposure to campaign messages, including in high-risk and underserved populations is also a concern. Finally, almost all assessed mass media campaigns have included multiple programme components (e.g. other community, school, and worksite interventions) and, therefore, the effects of mass media campaigns are difficult to isolate."[16] Involving other sectors of society in the healthcare campaign is an important part of their success.

LACK OF PHYSICAL ACTIVITY

A proper physical environment is a basic necessity for the success of a health physical fitness activity campaign. Not all open spaces in many communities are suitable for exercise and sports. There are requirements regarding a mapped-out area specific for exercise in Nigeria, like the National stadium, parks, game reserves, sports or recreational open fields. Some good institutions have standard play grounds and fields for exercise and sports. There is an issue with physical health environment at some urban schools, especially private schools in areas like Lagos which lack standard playgrounds for recreational activities. The problem is some pupils are deprived of proper physical exercise in schools, even during their daily break time or recreational sections. This has a negative effect on their body systems and mental capability when accumulated over time. Physical health fitness campaigns are set to address this issue.

According to the NIH, lack of environmental support (e.g., walking paths, like safety concerns, labor-saving products) is a competing influence affecting participants for physical fitness activities, of which its numbers and characteristics on mass media campaign in review are 19: ten community-wide for three mass media only, and six point-of-decision (Kahn et al, 2002). Then, 15 mass media campaigns with community programs (Cavill and Bauman, 2004), also 17 mass media with community programs (Finlay and Faulkner, 2005) another four mass media with community programs (Matson-Koffman et al, 2005) and five point-of-decision (Williams et al, 2008). The conclusion of the review states that there is moderate evidence for benefit on physical fitness activities, especially in motivated individuals and with prompts at their point of decision.[17]

Physical health was an ongoing campaign which was gaining public awareness but at some point, the campaign was dropped and physical activity started declining. However, with the help of concerned media and healthcare journalists to bring it back, a tremendously positive change in people's lifestyle and health fitness is being restored. More is expected for a complete compliance to prove the success of the campaign. The positive change will only be completely gained by the provision of equipment (e.g. gym apparatus, game facilities, etc.) and resource professionals (physicians, physical trainers, physio-therapists, nutritionists and more) which requires the involvement of the private sector.

"Health is wealth, participation in health related programmes though not compulsory but contribute greatly to all and development of the body and improve productivity [...] This will stem down the untimely deaths and incidences of cardiovascular diseases now common in Nigeria."[18] A physical health fitness campaign targets all ages who are healthy and fit enough to indulge in exercise. Of course, all individuals should follow the advice of their physicians on the type of fitness program in which to engage. Physical health campaigns seek to address nutritional values in connection to physical well-being as part of their agendas to transform individuals, group of people, and the society into productive active members of society. These campaigns are limited by the reality of non-availability of basic requirements for success including inadequate media campaign to enlighten members of the Nigerian community on the importance of exercise.

Nigeria National Policy on Education is one of the physical health campaigns in Nigeria that is currently functional, though it has not yet achieved complete success. "Today, physical education does not have the same prominence it once had and, in fact, the course is not taught in most Nigerian primary and secondary schools."[19] The media campaign on this policy has not yet achieved its purpose as not all schools adopted physical health education as a compulsory subject, even though "the National Policy on Education (Federal Republic of Nigeria 1977, 1981) was a document adopted by Nigeria's federal government to guide the administration and practice of education in the country. In this policy, the Nigerian government clearly stated that physical education would be emphasized at all levels of the educational system. These policy provisions tremendously helped [...] and made physical education a core subject in Nigeria's primary and secondary educational systems."[20]

The unfortunate fact is that most non-educated people assume that keeping fit is child's play or an activity that is a waste of time for adults to indulge. Recently, new programs on healthcare fitness involving people sharing testimonies of their new lifestyle and nutritional value change through the media campaigns prove that pure positive body response is achievable with physical fitness. This attracts more people to imitate and enroll in gymnastic clubs and other fitness activities promoting new active lifestyle in the society. These are evident on social media with pictures posted about ketogenics, iFitness, and others showing happy people whose body fitness has tremendously improved through the use of these approaches or devices.

"Campaigns with mass media components aimed at changing physical activity behaviours have yielded short-term increases in physical activity, mainly in highly motivated individuals. Success has been seen with community-wide walking campaigns targeting adults, especially older adults (e.g., >50 years), and the US Center for Disease Control and Prevention's VERB campaign, which targeted children aged 9–13 years. The latter campaign used commercial marketing techniques and had achieved population-level changes at year 2, with evidence being reported for an exposure-response relation."[21]

POOR NUTRITION

Media campaigns targeting poor nutrition are ongoing and the focus has always been to emphasize the importance of a balanced diet and the kinds of food nutrients being consumed as the foundation of a healthy lifestyle. Food, and more importantly its content, provides what our body needs to remain healthy. A balanced diet is highly recommended for all ages considering the state of the body and the activities to which we expose our bodies. It centers on people choosing to eat right over addictions.

The fight against poor nutrition is an on-going campaign. Its competing influences are food marketing and pricing which causes a severe hindrance for those encumbered by poverty. Lack of access to fresh fruit and vegetables is also a problem. The numbers and characteristics of its mass media campaigns in reviews are eight (Pomerleau et al, 2005), three communities and three labelling fruit and vegetables (Matson-Koffman et al, 2005) plus 29 point-of-purchase (Brownson et al, 2006). There is moderate evidence for benefit when specific healthy food choices are being promoted.[22]

Food promotions on media heightens awareness of the nutritional value that can be obtained from consuming it. Success of this communication depends on which particular nutrient is being promoted and the sources of food related to it. Then a choice must be made to promote a specific food with high concentrations of the desirable nutrient. The success of a media campaign on changing food consumption lifestyle of a particular community is relative to the food used for the campaign. For instance, when soya bean or soybean was promoted as a good source of protein on a media campaign, it popularized soya bean as food substance rich in protein making it very attractive and people consumed more soya bean during the campaign.

The issue of poor research by the campaigners serves to demote the success of media campaigns on poor nutrition. The media campaigners before embarking on liberating minds to new ideas and changing food consumption behavior of any community should perform comprehensive research on where to find the food item, the cost, how accessible is it for consumers, its nutritious value, and which the age range for which it is best recommended. The media campaign should educate the public on the consequences of lack of this nutrient in the body.

"Before 1990, campaigns related to diet frequently focused on reducing fat intake, but the results in terms of improving food choices seem to have been mixed. Later, media campaigns focused on increasing consumption of fruit, vegetables and low-fat milk, and were deemed more successful, especially when people were provided with access to healthy foods or had health disorders for which changes in diet would be beneficial."[23] Efforts to reduce fat intake is becoming increasingly popular as part of well-being maintenance. It should be noted that slim people often do not count themselves among those with high cholesterol, when realistically, cholesterol levels do not usually depend on the size of the individual. This is an area that needs additional focus as many people do not make this connection.

Fresh food, fruits or vegetables are more readily available in the rural areas. Those residing in some urban areas need information on the market and locations where these recommended foods can be found at reasonable prices. These markets must be easily accessible. Enlightening the public on overcoming transportation difficulties or the best routes to reach these market destinations is encouraged for positive compliance with healthy dietary needs. Farmers should be encouraged during such campaigns to increase the availability of the particular farm product and its substitutes. This requires research by the campaigners on the location of these rural farmers in the remote villages. Farmers who are not familiar with the farm product can be advised to try planting the crop as new crops/plants to serve their own community to curb scarcity although their success in this endeavor depends on the soil conditions in their environment. It requires advance notice and coordination with the farmers for the products to be ready during the campaign.

Convincing people to change their behavioral lifestyle is not an easy task but when all necessary aspects and requirements are put in place, positive compliance is obtainable. During a media campaign on poor nutrition, nutritionists along with traditional and medical doctors are recommended to participate in these campaigns. This set of professionals can provide advice on what to eat for people to obtain the essential nutrients their bodies need. These professionals, who are well-versed on detailed information about their particular subject are best prepared to answer questions during campaigns. Also, the target audience needs to be identified and located as part of planning the campaign.

Assessment of campaigns to promote nutrition and physical activity, compared to those promoting tobacco control, shows that while short-term changes can be achieved, sustained effects are difficult to maintain after campaigns end.[24]

CARDIOVASCULAR DISEASE PREVENTION

The WHO in summary states that cardiovascular disease is a major cause of disability and premature death throughout the world contributing substantially to the escalating costs of healthcare.[25] The underlying pathology is atherosclerosis which develops over many years and is usually advanced by the time symptoms occur, generally in middle age. Acute coronary and cerebrovascular events frequently occur suddenly, and are often fatal before medical care can be given.

Cardiovascular disease (CVD) Prevention is another constant campaign in relation to care for the heart, like exercising, keeping fit, and maintenance of body metabolism. The focus of the CVD Prevention media campaign is to encourage the modification of risk factors which aid in reducing the mortality and morbidity rate in a community. The human heart is certainly one of the main organs of the body that needs good care and maintenance to curb sudden death caused by breakdown or failure and loss of its function. Creating awareness through the media has been helpful in reducing disability and premature deaths from coronary heart disease, cerebrovascular disease, and peripheral vascular disease in people at high risk who have not yet experienced a cardiovascular event. The campaign guide is not recommended for people with established cardiovascular disease who are at very high risk of recurrent events.[26]

The WHO guidelines address individuals at high risk of CVD and encourage the practice of some forms of therapy that can prevent the reoccurrence of coronary, cerebral, and peripheral vascular events. There have been discussions on whether to introduce specific preventive actions, based on the degree of intensity and guided by an estimation of risk of a CVD attack. Risk prediction charts by the WHO offer instructions allowing treatment to be targeted according to simple predictions of absolute cardiovascular risk. Some recommendations are made for management of major cardiovascular risk factors through promotion of lifestyle change and the use of prophylactic drug therapies are encouraged. Associated media campaigns provide scope for the development of national guidance on prevention of cardiovascular disease that takes into account the particular political, economic, social, and medical circumstances.[27]

CVD is an on-going campaign and its competing influences are nutrition and physical activity and the numbers and characteristics of mass media campaigns in review for CVD prevention are five (Shea and Basch, 1990), five (Atienza and King, 2002) and seven community based (before 1998) with media components (Snyder et al, 2004). Nutrition is a concern in dealing with prevention and maintenance of CVD, and physical healthcare activities are highly encouraged for proper functioning of the heart as the power house of other organs of the body. Competitive influences imply that basic negative life-style results leading to CVD include poor nutrition and lack of physical activities. The summary and conclusions of the review states that there is moderate evidence for benefit in compliance.[28]

Lack of detailed information to back up contents used in campaigns for different sets of people grouped under diagnosed or undiagnosed cardiovascular disease prevention is hindering the success of the campaign. Those free from the disease require more of preventive practical measures. Each group needs their campaign content to provide sufficient detail on both preventive and maintenance life-style guidance. A significant proportion of morbidity and mortality could be prevented through population-based strategies, and by making cost-effective interventions accessible and affordable, both for people with established disease and for those at high risk of developing CVD.[29]

It is necessary to educate people on prevailing health problems and the methods of preventing and controlling them.[30] Media campaigns can become fruitless when campaigners on health issues of such high importance such as CVD are not equipped with basic knowledge and resources for enlightening the public on the prevalent risks of not adhering to the guides provided by health organizations or health officials and helping them adapt to new lifestyles suitable for a better livelihood. Campaigns are expected to tackle issues with evidence or proof on how effective the recommended healthcare techniques targeting CVD actually are. Evidence of how lives have been improved following past events of CVD is recommended for gaining audience attention during media campaigns. Testimonies of peoples' positive experiences while adapting to new life-styles is useful in capturing audience attention for compliance and providing continued encouragement during campaigns.

The challenge of providing valid information has always been the issue on providing content for healthcare in Nigeria. "Adediji says the information flow has been really bad and people have not been properly educated."[31] Poor information flow is noticed when people disbelieve guidance or healthcare recommendations. When the target audience ignores or rejects campaign instructions, it could be as a result of rumors which might be prompted by fear of the unknown on issues like rejecting medications prescribed for disease prevention. It is essential to provide health workers the information that proves the prescribed medications are safe for them before they can be expected to administer them to others. The outcome of the tests associated with the use of these medications on medical officials helps prove they will be safe for members of the general population.

BIRTH RATE REDUCTION

"In 1950, women were having an average of 4.7 children in their lifetime. Researchers at the University of Washington's Institute for Health Metrics and Evaluation showed the global fertility rate nearly halved to 2.4 in 2017 - and their study, published in the Lancet, projects it will fall below 1.7 by 2100."[32]

This research is based on the fact that the fertility rate is measured by the average number of children to which a woman gives birth. As the fertility rate falls then the size of the population also decreases. In 1950, women were having an average of 4.7 children in their lifetime. This is almost half of the rate currently being recorded.

Efforts to reduce the birthrate represent an on-going campaign, which has the competing influences of social norms for family size and lack of access to relevant services. Social norm here means the cultural beliefs that contribute to birth rate and family size, particularly, the number of children in each family which ultimately drives the total population of a community. The numbers and characteristics of mass media campaigns in reviews are 15 (Hornik and McAnany, 2001). This review concludes that there is moderate evidence for benefit from the campaign, especially among motivated individuals.[33]

A campaign of this nature requires a good presentation with drawings and figures covering a full range of the target populations with proper documentation and pictures to provide systematic evidence for capturing their interest. Poor presentation of the information distorts the works of researchers and can mar the success of the campaign. A systematic presentation provides evidence on the detailed research and its usefulness which is very necessary for sharing the information in a convincing manner. In the African community, pictures serve better in presentations to provide a quick demonstration of what is rejected, its causes and effects as well as what is acceptable along with its benefits.

Successful measures used by other communities in achieving compliance can help as evidence of a successful campaign targeting birth rate control. For example, family planning practices that are acceptable in the western world could serve as a positive reinforcement for local or regional campaigns. "Those intended to encourage family planning have been particularly important in low-income countries. The transition from high to low birth rates has been argued to require a climate of opinion 'supportive of modern contraceptive use and the idea of smaller family sizes.'"[34] This opinion is supported by substantial evidence that the spread of information through mass media, along with efforts to promote family planning, is associated with adoption of contraception. Positive outcomes can be shown whether comparisons are made across geographic areas, over time within geographic areas, or between individuals.

Evidence proves that effective birth rate reduction is gaining positive response with family planning communication strategies being embedded as pro-family planning messages in entertainment programs such as music, soap operas, social gatherings, and focused advertising. "The greatest short-term increases in demand have been reported for people who were exposed to campaign messages and were already considering use; the effects in people who were not previously committed to use are less convincing."[35]

HIV INFECTION PREVENTION

One of the most popular healthcare media campaigns is Human Immunodeficiency Virus (HIV) Infection Prevention. The devastation experienced by affected individuals and the risks of unhealthy lifestyles serve in garnering the attention of the public about the dangers or this disease. The high death rate reported in HIV cases around the world proves its existence and serves as a cautionary measure for people who may doubt its existence. Some HIV patients also prove how horrible the dreadful disease can be on humans.

HIV Infection Prevention is an ongoing campaign and its competing influences are human sexual drive, cultural reinforcement of risky behaviors, and lack of access to services. The numbers and characteristics of mass media campaign in review are eight (Wellings, 2002), 24 (Bertrand et al, 2006) and 34 complementary to other interventions and routine media coverage of AIDS (Noar et al, 2009). The conclusion of this review states that there is moderate evidence for benefit on condom use and little evidence for benefit associated with the number of sex partners.[36]

A successful media campaign on HIV Infection Prevention is determined by certain factors including the strategic technique applied, government policies, motivation, social norm and culture, duration, and education. Good planning and strategic technique application are key to a successful HIV campaign. Government and health organizations can work together on the policy provision as a recommended guide with penalties for those who do not adhere to the new norm. The target audience are motivated for change with the benefits attached to the new norm compliance and policies. However, they are controlled by their environmental coexistence with others regarding their old ways of livelihood and culture. Adapting to the new ways of life will take time and requires patience. The level of education of individuals in a community also determines how quickly and well they can understand and accept any healthcare campaign instructions. If consideration is given to these issues, HIV Infection Prevention media campaigns will achieve increased positive results in terms of credibility and compliance.[37]

Obstacles hindering successful HIV Prevention media campaigns are opposing messages shared by pervasive and competitive marketing of products recommended to prevent the infection, social norm, addiction, long-term and short-term duration, cluttered media environment, lack of strategic planning and practical tests on campaign contents, and formats or products with the right target audience. Most companies producing the materials or medications used in prevention of HIV infection are involved in a highly competitive market. They tend to promote their products and demote their competitors with negative comments that can cause distractions and confusion in the public sphere. Social norms affect campaigns when the new norm is not aligning with the cultural behavior of the people in a community. For example, the use of sharp objects associated with female circumcision. Habitual behaviors are risky and create a huge problem considering the long-term goal of obtaining positive change. Planning requires creative strategies and the environmental factor often presents a challenge for a successful campaign. Testing of the recommended content on the right target group is a good technique that should always be considered in planning a campaign on HIV infection prevention.[38]

CERVICAL CANCER SCREENING AND PREVENTION

Cervical cancer is a type of cancer associated with women's cervix and reproductive organs. It is a leading cause of cancer among females in the developing world. A survey of 483 randomly selected Nigerian women at Aleshinloye Market conducted by questionnaire in November, 2003, probed into their sexual history, awareness about cervical cancer, and the extent of utilization of Pap smear. Results showed that the majority (79.5%) of the women were sexually active. One hundred and eighty-six (38.5%) had early sexual encounters and 163 (33.7%) had multiple sexual partners. Of the population surveyed, only 197 respondents (40.8%) were aware of cervical cancer. Of these, 95 (19.7%) were aware of the Papanicolaou (Pap) smears as a screening test. The common means of awareness among those surveyed included by radio and television (46.6%), public lecture (27.8%), and friends or relatives (19.9%). However, only 25 respondents (5.2%) had been tested with a Pap smear.[39]

A report produced as a result of the survey concluded that "though the market women are at considerable risk of developing cancer of the cervix, they are poorly informed about the disease and its prevention. Therefore, there is need for continuous awareness campaign and well-organized screening programs among this unique category of women."[40]

The Cervical Cancer Screening and Prevention campaign targets an episodic type of behavioral change that requires diagnosis and screening. Its competition influence is lack of access to screening services in most rural regions. The numbers and characteristics of mass media campaigns in reviews for cervical cancer are ten: four mass media alone, six with other components (Black et al 2002), and three mass media alone (Baron et al 2008). There is moderate evidence of benefit when used with other programs in expanding the impact of the campaign.[41]

Mass media campaigns aim at encouraging women to have Pap smears and undergo screening. Mammography, a technique using X-rays to diagnose and locate tumors of the breasts, have been run in many high-income nations since the early 1990s. "Initial experience, predominantly from Australia and the USA, suggested that mass media campaigns supported by tailored reminder letters prompted short-term increases in Pap smear uptake, especially when there was good availability of screening services. Later research indicated that short-duration screening programmes that offered easy access to screening services, used reminder letters, and specifically included television broadcast components were associated with short-term population-wide increases in attendance for Pap smears, including in ethnic minority population and those of low socioeconomic status."[42]

Campaigns based in the US and findings in cases of mammography suggests a small but significant effect. Areas where screening was already organized and available led to increase in uptake claimed by L. B. Snyder and colleagues in their article entitled "A meta-analysis of the effect of mediated health communication campaigns on behavior change in the United States" in 2004 using their meta-analysis. Mass media campaigns without organized screening services, produced little or no detectable increases in use of cervical cancer screening. A systematic review proves insufficient evidence of an association between mass media campaigns alone even when accompanied by comprehensive community programs and changes in exposure to sunlight behaviors.[43]

Lack of trained media persons in carrying out a particular health task during campaign especially on issues concerning screening, like the case of cervical cancer screening and prevention is a huge task for campaign planners in Nigeria. It deals with interest and exposure to healthcare trainings to perform better as a functional and practical media campaigner. Some questions demand instant feedback and during campaigns, such questions are expected to be handled instantly by the campaigners. There is need for technical knowledge on how the health equipment for screening works. This requires training and technical knowledge, though with patience for experts who can handle it to manifest among selected media campaigners.

Some rural areas have less expertise in this area compared to health professionals in urban areas. Most Nigerians in the rural parts of the country must travel some distance to access the screening centers. Transportation costs are so high that interest in obtaining screenings often lost which increases stress for those women. Campaigns not only serve to create awareness but basic necessities required for its success must be taken into consideration in order for the campaigns to achieve positive results. The screening centers which are currently available are not sufficient leaving women in the rural parts of Nigeria underserved.

BREAST CANCER SCREENING AND PREVENTION

"Breast cancer is a major killer of women both globally and regionally. Studies have shown that most patients with breast cancer in the Eastern Mediterranean Region present for the first time at stages two and three, indicating the need for increased community awareness and early detection of the disease. Well-conceived and well managed national cancer control programmes are able to lower cancer incidence and improve the lives of people living with cancer. These evidence-base and guidelines have been designed to support Ministries of Health in their policy-setting for early detection and screening of breast cancer, as well as to assist health care providers and patients in decision-making in the most commonly encountered situations."[44] Breast cancer is a time-bound disease that when neglected or if not detected early enough claims the lives of too many women. Knowledge of the symptoms is a key factor for early detection.

"In developing countries, the majority of women diagnosed with breast cancer do not survive because their cancer is detected too late. Motunrayo Bello reports on the challenges of dealing with breast cancer in Nigeria."[45]

Breast cancer screening is an episodic type of behavioral change campaign and its competing influence is lack of access to screening services. The numbers and characteristics of mass media campaigns in reviews are four with community programs (Snyder et al, 2004) and zero that were mass media only (Baron et al, 2008). The review reported that there was moderate evidence of benefit when mass media campaigns were combined with community programs but no findings for campaigns the used mass media only.[46]

The success or failure of these programs have so much to do with people's belief and religion. One of the major barriers of this campaign is the fact that breasts are considered a private part of a woman's body. The clinical breast exam (CBE) acceptance is low and seeking the opinion of the target population is handicapped. "Approximately 99% of women respondents in our study ascribed to some religious affiliation. It is encouraging that more than two thirds of the respondents were willing to have regular CBEs. Responses from women who declined such examination suggest that with proper education and awareness, many more women are likely to be won over, given that the reasons for non-willingness were related to lack of perceived need."[47]

According to the WHO, "so far the only breast cancer screening method that has proved to be effective is mammography screening."[48] "In limited resource settings with weak health systems, organized population-based mammography screening programs may not be cost-effective and feasible. Early diagnosis of symptomatic women with prompt diagnosis and treatment should be the priority. In these settings, clinical breast examination, seems to be a promising screening approach."[49] This is one of the most popular cancer campaigns in Nigeria. Since many social norms surround the issues associated with a breast cancer campaign and self-detection as well as screening tests, the success of such efforts has a lot to do with education and increasing awareness among women.

BOWEL CANCER SCREENING AND PREVENTION

Bowel cancer can start in the large bowel (colon) or the back passage (rectum). It is also known as colorectal cancer. Bowel cancer is divided into different types depending on where it starts in the bowel, and the type of cell in which it starts.

Bowel Cancer Screening and Prevention is an episodic type of behavioral campaign. Its competing influence is lack of access to screening services. The number and characteristics of mass media campaigns in reviews is zero, which were mass media only (Baron et al, 2008). The summary indicates that there is no evidence for mass media.[50] This implies that bowel cancer needs media sensitization of the dreadful disease to make impact in the behavioral change expected for its prevention. When there is no mass media campaign on Bowel cancer, an expectation of compliance cannot be achieved because a mass media would offer a strong channel to create awareness and show seriousness in disseminating information.

"Cancer Council Australia calls for extended Government investment to continue to increase screening program participation. New research released [...] has highlighted the lifesaving potential of promoting bowel cancer screening, showing that a national four-year awareness campaign could prompt over one million Australians to participate in the screening program and save 4330 Australian lives over the next 40 years. The modelling, conducted by Cancer Council NSW [New South Wales] and published in the journal Public Health, also shows that a four-year national campaign could prevent 8100 bowel cancer cases. The release of the new research coincides with data released by the Australian Institute of Health and Welfare [...] showing that only 42% of eligible Australians took part."[51]

A Nigerian study has proven that screening for colorectal cancer (CRC) is effective in reducing disease mortality and it is also cost effective. It was discovered that recent reports on colorectal cancer are common in Nigeria. The results of the study indicate that there were "300 respondents with a mean age (SD) of 33 (7.8) years and an age range of 23 - 67 years. In terms of duration of medical practice, 190 (63%) were short, 43 (14%) medium and 67 (23%) long. Majority (65%) of the respondents were in teaching hospitals, 18.5% in private hospitals and 5.7% were in general (community) hospitals. The knowledge of the clinical features as well as the risk factors of CRC was fair in over 75% of the respondents. Most respondents, 265 (87.8%), agreed that CRC was worth screening for; 21 (5%) did not. In all, 246 (82%) gave reasons for their responses. However, just over half of the respondents employed one of the following: fecal occult blood test (FOBT), double contrast barium enema (DCBE), flexible sigmoidoscopy, colonoscopy, or a combination of any of the techniques for screening. Usage of CT colonography was low. Screening rates by respondents for other malignancies in this survey was higher than that of CRC (prostate 95%, breast 97%, cervix 99%)."[52]

The study concluded that the awareness of CRC screening is high, though its performance is very low and highly valuable in form. The study suggests that there is need for improved practice of CRC screening through sensitizing of medical practitioners to effectively provide all diagnosis resources and effective local guidelines.[53] When compared to breast cancer awareness in Nigeria, bowel cancer (colorectal cancer) is not yet as well publicized as breast cancer sensitization in Nigeria. Although the media campaign, as stated in the study, proved effective, its performance is still very low. However, it is not about awareness alone but the practical response it produces within a population that is essential for the ultimate success of the campaign.

The accessibility screening centers is an issue connected to all cancer media campaign compliance in Nigeria by the citizens. People need guidance on recognizing the symptoms of bowel cancer to enable them to identify the disease in its early stages at homes. Campaign participants need to be equipped with the facts, well-researched information on preventive measures, and early diagnostic details on cancerous diseases in order for them to be able to offer convincing approaches that guide behavioral change. Personal evidence and proof-of-life experience serves best in converting individuals to self-examining habits for identifying indications of bowel cancer and all cancerous diseases.

SKIN CANCER PREVENTION

Mass media campaigns aim at preventing skin cancer and its focus is on reducing patterns of sun exposure on the skin, mainly in fair-skinned populations. There are recommendations on the expected behavioral change which includes avoidance of direct exposure to sunlight in high ultraviolet periods, wearing protective clothing materials, and using sunscreen products to protect the skin from direct sunlight, since skin cancer is caused mainly by overexposure to ultraviolet radiation in sunlight. Screening of asymptomatic individuals for skin cancer is also recommended for early detection of squamous cell cancer (SCC), basal cell cancer (BCC), and malignant melanoma.

Skin cancer prevention is an on-going behavioral media campaign and its competing influence is the social norm for tanning. Numbers and characteristics of mass media campaigns in reviews on skin cancer are 47: 12 mass media only, 35 with community interventions (Saraiya et al, 2004). The review states that there is insufficient evidence for individual behavioral change associated with skin cancer prevention.[54]

Research from Australia assessed sun protection attitudes and behaviors for 15 years in the presence of variable amounts of media campaign exposure. It proved that there have been improvements in behavioral change associated with skin cancer prevention as a result of media campaigns. It was also discovered that there was a reduction of melanoma observed among young people over the decades of the media campaign. These researchers advocate for sustained community-wide organized efforts that include mass media to maintain the positive preventive effects and to counter competing forces that encourage sunbathing and tanning as well as fashion trends and marketing that promote some types of clothing materials from luxury designers, that promote class identification, which are not suitable under excessive sunlight and solarium marketing.[55]

Weather is an important factor to consider. Africa is a hot region and Africans are adaptable to sunlight because of their skin type due to the amount of melanin they have in their skin. When a light-skinned person decides to tan the skin, sunscreen is advised to reduce the negative effects of direct sunlight.

IMPROVED IMMUNIZATION

Sensitization to the importance of improved immunization is one of the most popular media campaigns in Nigeria. Mothers are concerned with the health and welfare of their babies and this has contributed to the levels of compliance observed over the years since the inception of immunization campaign and awareness. There are basic hindrances reducing the level of compliance expected such as the high level of illiteracy but antenatal programs for pregnant women in Nigeria promote awareness of the importance of immunization as a support system which is gaining ground in improving healthcare.

A Bangladesh review on immunization behavioral change found four of six childhood vaccination programs that used mass media to achieve a substantial improvement in vaccine use. The effects were incremental with increasing exposure to the campaign. The cost-effectiveness analysis attributed to the increase in the use of immunization services to national campaign awareness. No additional examples of mass media campaigns were found by a later review on vaccination interventions. Mass media was a strategy widely adopted in multi-component vaccination campaigns worldwide. It was observed that substantial improvements in childhood vaccination were repeatedly recorded. The effectiveness of improved immunization sensitization is not specifically attached to mass media campaigns.[56]

Improved immunization media campaign is a one-time or episodic type of behavioral change. Lack of access to vaccine is its competing influence. The numbers and characteristics of mass media campaigns in review for immunization sensitization are seven complementing improved vaccination access (Hornik et al, 2002) and four mass media (Pegurri et al, 2005). The conclusion of the review states that there is moderate evidence for benefit from the campaign.[57]

The WHO reported on November 16, 2019, that efforts continued boosting the immunity of children against measles and meningitis. The government of Nigeria through the National Primary Health Care Development Agency (NPHCDA) in conjunction with the WHO and support from Gavi, the Vaccine Alliance, launched a largescale campaign to reach more than 28 million children with lifesaving vaccines. "Government is committed to ensuring every eligible child is reached with these lifesaving vaccines. We will go to markets, schools, churches, mosques and everywhere we can get good catchment to reach our target population. No child deserves to die from any vaccine preventable disease." Dr. Joseph Oteri, Director of Disease Control and Immunization, NPHCDA. These children are set to be vaccinated across 19 northern Nigerian states, namely: Bauchi, Benue, Borno, Kano, Katsina, Plateau, Taraba, Niger, Adamawa, Kaduna, and Sokoto as well as other states including Gombe Jigawa, Kebbi, Nasarawa, Yobe, Zamfara, Kwara, and the Federal Capital Territory.[58]

DIARRHEA DISEASE PREVENTION

The campaign to prevent diarrhea is a popular media awareness that promotes childcare with the available vaccination given to babies along with immunizations for other diseases. The key measures to prevent diarrhea are access to safe drinking water, use of improved sanitation, hand washing with soap, exclusive breastfeeding for the first six months of life, good personal and food hygiene, health education about how infections spread, and rotavirus vaccination.[59] "Five diarrhoea treatment programmes that used mass media to promote home-mixed or premixed rehydration solutions, three were associated with increased adoption of rehydration solution."[60]

Diarrhea is a type of behavioral disease campaign that is episodic and its competing influence is previous custom of withdrawing food and liquids while feeding new-born babies. The numbers and characteristics of mass media campaigns in review on diarrhea are five with improved access to premixed rehydration solution and health-worker training (Hornik et al, 2002). Results indicate moderate evidence for benefit from the campaign.[61]

"In July 2019, the World Health Organization set the global norm to deploy a simple, powerful game-changer: the ORS + zinc co-pack." The diarrhea campaign encourages mothers to administer an oral rehydration solution (ORS) as a simple treatment easy to prepare with a mixture of salt, water and sugar. The ORS provides first aid and quick recovery treatment, if well managed. The Lancet has called ORS one of the most important medical advances of the twentieth century.[62]

Important information that should be properly discussed in detail during campaigns includes messages such as zinc is an essential nutrient that becomes depleted during diarrhea. Administering a supplement reduces the duration of diarrhea and prevents future episodes. A global recommendation to formalize use of the ORS and zinc co-pack as the gold standard treatment for diarrhea in 2004 was set up by the WHO.[63] When mothers are well informed with facts concerning the dangers if diarrhea is not well-managed and properly handled, they will generally adopt the recommended techniques required for saving the lives of their babies.

INCREASED BREASTFEEDING

The campaign on increased breastfeeding in Nigeria is still ongoing and mothers are advised to practice exclusive breast feeding to promote the breastmilk from mother-to-child consumption. A Nigerian study on Impact Assessment of Exclusive Breastfeeding Media Campaign Among Mothers in Selected Metropolitan Cities in South East Nigeria claims that the mass media by virtue of disseminating information plays a vital role in communication for health and sustainable development of the society. This study examines the impact of the exclusive breastfeeding media campaigns targeting mothers in selected metropolitan cities in South East Nigeria to ascertain their disposition to exclusive breastfeeding using media campaign messages.[64]

The Increase Breastfeeding campaign is a one-off or episodic campaign and its competing influences are cultural preferences and hospital practices. The numbers and characteristics of mass media campaigns in reviews are two with health-worker retraining (McDivitt et al, 1993) and three with health-worker retraining or restricted marketing of infant formula (Wilmoth and Elder, 1995). The conclusion states that the evidence for benefit on the campaign is weak.[65]

"Breastfeeding is encouraged at any point in time be it, in the open / public or in isolation. The belief of Africans is that breastfeeding is an ingredient of promotion of closeness to mothers and a concept of bringing the mother and child closer to one another. It is even seen as taboo for a mother not to breastfeed her child."[66] The issue with breastfeeding is with the new generation mothers who follow a fashion trend that hinders their babies from accessing their breast when out of their homes. The belief of breastfeeding as the reason behind breast sagging among women is another factor contributing to the non-compliance of some mothers to the breastfeeding campaign.

The study observed that some factors are responsible for its effectiveness among women. These factors include but are not limited to ignorance and lack of education. With the use of qualitative and quantitative mixed research approaches, the findings reveal evidence of the positive impact of exclusive breastfeeding media campaign messages on mothers in South East Nigeria. The study points to the fact that antenatal is still a major platform for educating women on breastfeeding for a successful campaign compared to media channels in the region. The study states that "much more is still required from the traditional media platforms especially in terms of enlivened programme design and committed publicity to rightly occupy their place in this campaign role considering the heterogeneous nature of the audience they serve, which predisposes them more advantageous to reach even prospective mothers (those not yet expecting babies) who may not have immediate need to come for antenatal to access such beneficial nutritional and health information."[67]

"Although mass media programmes to promote breastfeeding have been mounted, reviews from the 1990s onwards seem scarce or non-existent. Two studies—one from Jordan in the late 1980s and one from Armenia show positive effects."[68]

IMPROVED ROAD SAFETY

The campaign to improve road safety is ongoing but more frequently implemented during festive seasons and is often accompanied by government policies in checkmating public attitudes on road use by addressing the concern drivers have for their own lives and the lives of others while driving. Road safety officials give direct instructions to road users which promotes compliance and positive attitude of drivers. "The mass media campaigns on road use by road safety aid in reducing death rate with the cautioning on use of seatbelts, booster seats for children, and helmets for bicyclists, skateboarders, motorcyclists, reductions in speeding, driver fatigue, and drink driving cautions."[69]

Improved Road Safety is an ongoing behavioral campaign and its competing influences are alcohol marketing and pricing, drowsiness, and road and vehicle designs. The Numbers and characteristics of mass media campaigns in its reviews are 15 with enforcement campaigns (Dinh-Zarr et al, 2001), 87 and 35 with other campaigns for road safety and comparison groups (Morrison, et al, 2003) also Nine (Ditter et al, 2005) and Eight with campaigns for drunk-driving (Elder et al, 2004). Studies on this topic conclude that there is strong evidence for increased use of safety belts and decreased drunk driving when enforcement campaigns are used, and there are mixed conclusions for designated driver campaigns on road safety.[70]

"The average associated decline in vehicle crashes has been estimated to be at least 7%, and of alcohol-impaired driving to be 13%. Results of designated driver programmes have been less conclusive. The most notable road safety campaigns have promoted seat belt use. The Click It or Ticket programme in North Carolina, USA, was associated with an increase in seat belt use from 63% to 80% and lowered rates of highway deaths, and became a model for other state and national programmes. A version in Washington state, USA, reported gains from 83% up to 95% of seat belt use. Law enforcement and repeated cycles of short-term mass media exposure seem, therefore, to have been important components of road safety campaign effectiveness."[71]

Some nongovernmental organization (NGO) programs such as the "Light Up the Night for Traffic Safety" is an initiative of the NGO alliance member Safety Beyond Boarders, formerly Safety Alliance, in Nigeria. The program instructs and mobilizes Nigerians to use a pair of 45-centimeter-long reflective straps or tapes to promote the visibility of their vehicles when traveling on the road at night. Car owners and drivers of large vehicles including trucks, petrol tankers, and trailers are requested to stick these reflective tapes on their vehicles so they can be seen from a distance of about 500 meters by other road users. This aids in preventing traffic accidents.[72]

The aim of the campaign is to address the high incidence of road traffic crashes, injuries, and fatalities that occur across Nigerian roads at night, especially among long-distance travelers. Such long-distance travel causes a high occurrence of highway accidents and significant loss of life. Most highways in Nigeria are not lighted and lack road signs. Bad roads and the condition of vehicles, some of which some have no rear lights, contribute to the high rate of road accidents in Nigeria. Safety professionals embarked on a search for an affordable and effective solution. They studied the United States reflective straps in the safety of road users at night and as a result created the Light Up the Night for Traffic Safety initiative in Nigeria. The campaign commenced in 2002-2003 with Lagos State as its pilot location. The scope of the program has since expanded. The team extended their efforts to include the of placing reflective tape on the roads in blind spots and high-risk areas and conduct systematic monitoring of blind spots.[73]

"Comparing the incidence of night crashes before the campaign was launched to after the campaign roll-out. The findings are encouraging. For example, the crash rate at one blind spot located on the Third Mainland Bridge was reduced by over 92%—from an average of five crashes per month to one or two in five to six months."[74] The observation proved that there is reduction difference in traffic crashes and resulting injuries and fatalities across Nigeria since the inception of the program. "Most drivers surveyed agreed that reflective tapes have drastically improved visibility during the night. Of the 500 polled vehicle owners and drivers, 85% stated that they can more clearly and quickly see vehicles with reflective tapes than vehicles without these devices when they are driving on the roads."[75]

INCREASED ORGAN DONATION

The Increased Organ Donation campaign requires well-informed people to carry out the proper measures for educating the public on the details and laws attached to the donation of body parts. There are a lot of misconceptions and beliefs associated with organ donation. Many public hospitals across Nigeria are involved in kidney transplantation. The laws must be applied while carrying out such a serious act to protect the medical officials practicing it and to prevent them from becoming victims of abuse. "Majority of these centers carry out few transplantations in a year and months apart. This is tantamount to the dissipation of limited resources and energy. The existing transplant centers in the country could be merged into regional centers. Such regional centers should be funded sufficiently by the government to have adequate facilities for transplantation."[76]

Increased organ donation is a type of behavioral change campaign that takes place as one-off events. Its competing influences are cultural, religious beliefs and family relationships. The numbers and characteristics of its mass media campaign in review are 14 complementing World Transplant Games Federation events (Slapak, 2004). Reviews indicate that there is moderate evidence showing the benefit on this campaign.[77]

Organ transplantation is globally becoming a popular concern. It is not supported by a regular campaign. Based on an assessment of organ donations, mixed results have been observed. Public misconceptions and mistrust surrounding end-of-life decisions by physicians creates a barrier to change as expected of the campaign. With few publications on blood donation, some studies do report a sizeable increase in blood donors in conjunction to mass media campaigns. "For example, during China's national campaign to promote safe donation, which used celebrities and a patriotic message, the number of voluntary blood donors rose from 55 to 96, 320 in one city between 1993 and 2001. 91 in Ghana, analysis of a low-cost radio campaign that promoted voluntary blood donation from 2003 to 2006 showed an associated high response from young male donors attending for repeat donation who had not previously done so."[78]

The major common challenge of organ donation is shortage of organs from willing living donors. Kidney transplant in Nigeria is low and remains an issue even with the advanced techniques that have been developed to ensure the success of organ transplants.[79]

"Direct payment for donated organ have been admitted to be unethical worldwide and widely condemned by many countries. Although, there is a formal condemnation of payment for organs, the markets actually thrive, especially, as a significant component of transplant tourism. Unfortunately, altruistic donations have not been sufficient to take care of patients with ERSD on the waiting list. In the USA, about 17 patients died each day while waiting to be transplanted."[80]

IMPROVED MENTAL HEALTH AND REDUCED VIOLENCE AND CHILD MALTREATMENT

The expected behavioral change for Mental Health and Reduced Violence and Child Maltreatment campaign is the rate of child abuse and maltreatment recorded. "Child abuse or maltreatment constitutes all forms of physical and/or emotional ill-treatment, sexual abuse, neglect or negligent treatment or commercial or other exploitation, resulting in actual or potential harm to the child's health, survival, development or dignity in the context of a relationship of responsibility, trust or power."[81] This definition was drafted by the WHO in 1999.

The various forms of child abuse and maltreatment perpetrates violence against children and promotes mental disorder among children. The International Society for the Prevention of Child Abuse and Neglect recently compared definitions of abuse from 58 countries and found some commonality in what was considered abusive. The four types of abuses observed were physical abuse, sexual abuse, emotional abuse, and neglect.[82]

Mental Health Violence and Child Maltreatment is an on-going behavioral change campaign and its competing influences are social norms and access to violent means of harm (weapons, drugs, etcetera). The numbers and characteristics of mass media campaigns in reviews are five (Mikton and Butchert, 2009) and five (Mann et al, 2005). It concludes that the campaign results provide inconclusive findings for behavior changes in child maltreatment and little evidence for benefit in suicide prevention.[83]

Some sources from the Centers for Disease Control and Prevention and the WHO claim that youth violence, intimate partner violence, child maltreatment of both sexual and physical abuse, and mental disorders are preventable behaviors with negative effects on high rates of injuries and deaths, including physical health conditions. Researchers seek mass media interventions to redress risk factors. Examples of promising programs with mass media components include a campaign for professional training that lowered rates of child maltreatment results. Another is an intimate partner violence program for which increased bystander responses were reported as well as a campaign that was associated with reduced rates of bullying in schools among children aged 12 to 14 years of age.[84]

Regarding the abusive treatment resulting in suicide among victims, a review of suicide prevention campaigns undertaken in several countries found improvements in attitudes about causes and treatment of depression but outcomes such as the rate of suicide acts did not change.[85] This has a lot to do with the extent to which child maltreatment or any form of abuse effects human mental processes leading to self-termination of lives.

"Documentation of effective responses, relatively few studies have been carried out on the effectiveness of responses to prevent child abuse and neglect. There is thus an urgent need, in both industrialized and developing countries, for the rigorous evaluation of many of the preventive responses described above. Other existing interventions should also be assessed with regard to their potential for preventing abuse – for instance, child support payments, paid paternity and maternity leave, and early childhood programmes."[86]

There is need for more research investigating cultural differences and acceptance on forms of disciplinary behaviors in various cultures around the world. This will provide information on expectations and choices of parents raising their children in a particular region. Abuse as a dangerous health issue for children ought to be tackled from the root causes considering the general acceptance of some cultural disciplinary practices. This is achievable if researchers are determined to explore further on reaching a broader consensus on the detrimental impact of employing harsh disciplinary acts on children.

The issue of neglect demands some forms of investigation on the status of the family of the abused child. It is important to discover how best to distinguish neglect by parents from deprivation through poverty and intentional abuse by torturing a child. The victims of abuse are mostly identified among the low-income earners and low-educated or non-educated individuals.

To achieve compliance, new approaches are needed which must be tested regarding their influence on primary prevention as well as improved training and education. It is the responsibility of educational health professionals to design new approaches to child abuse positive response through media campaigns. Researchers in the fields of medicine and public health are obliged to skillfully design and conduct investigations of abuse perpetrated in public and in homes. More is expected of the social and behavioral scientists, and teachers using the training programs including the subject of child abuse and the development within organizations in contribution to school curriculum.

Legal provisions are necessary to aid quell disciplinary abusive acts in the society. "In Europe, Poland is one of the countries that have integrated the stipulations of the Convention into their domestic law. Local government bodies in that country now have a responsibility to provide social, psychiatric and legal aid for children. In Africa, Ghana has also amended its criminal code, raised the penalties for rape and molestation, and abolished the option of fines for offences involving sexual violence. The government has also conducted educational campaigns on issues relating to the rights of children, including child abuse. Only a few countries, though, have legal provisions covering all forms of violence against children."[87]

IMPROVED PREHOSPITAL RESPONSE TIMES FOR POTENTIAL HEART ATTACK SYMPTOMS

Heart disease is a dangerous disease that catches people unaware and steals lives. The campaign for Improved Prehospital Response Times for Potential Heart Attack Symptoms in Nigeria is raising the alarm on the importance of quick governmental intervention to provide aid in addressing the issue. This will require active citizen awareness to curb the ravaging sudden death counts recorded in the country. "In June 2016, Stephen Keshi, former Super Eagles head coach, died at age 58 of a suspected cardiac arrest. Four days later, Shuaibu Amodu, another former Super Eagles coach, was found dead in his bed, aged 54, after complaining of chest pains the night before. There are countless stories of other young Nigerians who have just apparently 'slumped and died.' These stories all affirm a growing epidemic of heart disease in Nigeria and other low and middle-income countries."[88]

Improved Prehospital Response Times for Potential Heart Attack Symptoms is an episodic type of behavioral change campaign. Its competing influences are rural location and failure to recognize severity of the disease symptoms in the body system. The numbers and characteristics of mass media campaigns in reviews on it are 16 with other components (Finn et al, 2007). The conclusion states that there is moderate evidence for decreased delay and emergency calls on the expected compliance to the campaign.[89]

"Mass media campaigns to reduce delays in prehospital response for heart attacks and other emergency health disorders have been related to increased understanding of symptoms but no sustained lowering of response times or mortality rates. Researchers have called for extension of campaign duration to increase exposure, and strengthening of the messages by concurrently offering community programmes, targeting of high-risk and rural populations, and investigation of patients' barriers to action."[90]

The data from the WHO indicates that "over half a million Nigerians died from non-communicable diseases (NCDs) in 2012, and one out of every five Nigerian adults over the age of 30 will likely die prematurely from NCDs, including cardiovascular diseases. In terms of risk factors for heart disease, 35% of Nigerian adults had elevated blood pressures in 2008, another 6.5%, mostly women, were obese."[91]

"Although the Nigerian Tobacco Control Act was signed into action in 2015, several of its provisions were too weak and its implementation in Nigeria by the Federal Ministry of Health has been lacking. The ban on smoking in public places needs to be enforced, taxation on tobacco products needs to be increased, and other provisions of the Framework Convention on Tobacco Control (FCTC) to which Nigeria signed in 2006 need to be enforced."[92] Disciplining smokers to avoid public places while smoking requires serious follow-up and consequences for violations of the law. This will help enhance the impact of the media campaign to yield positive results.

Recommendations

These recommendations serve as processes to be recognized in correcting issues in connection to social problems targeted with media campaigns.

GOVERNMENT AGENCIES IN CONJUNCTION WITH HEALTH ORGANIZATIONS AND OTHER POLICY MAKING BODIES

The Government agencies and their policy-making bodies play a significant role in supporting behavioral change with high expectation for positive outcomes. When government policy is aligned with behavioral change campaigns, compliance is greatly improved. This is based on the fact that penalties have been created to limit noncompliance. The high percentage of public response to government healthcare policies in conjunction with health organizations recommendations is a commendable and recommended approach to compliance on certain healthcare media campaigns.

Nigerian media largely depends on the WHO and other global health organizations for information on healthcare as much as a child in the womb depends on his mother to survive. There is a high tendency for healthcare information generated from the WHO to be generally accepted as a reliable source of information by the public. Hearing directly from a credible source such as the WHO can be convincing and makes the information provided in a publication more credible and authentic.

This makes perfect sense since the WHO is a global body designed to fight and control diseases. An example is Communication for Behavioral Impact (COMBI), a program with a toolkit recommended by the WHO, which has a planning framework and integrates behavioral and social communication interventions within public health programs. The COMBI toolkit is an important example of a fundamental shift in how the public comprehends and complies by application of communicable disease outbreak control techniques as in the case of Ebola in 2014. The ability to shift human behavior is a major factor determining the risk for the spread of diseases with epidemic potential.

REGULATIONS ON SOCIAL MEDIA TO REDUCE MISGUIDANCE, SOCIAL NORMS, AND BELIEFS AFFECTING THE FUNCTIONALITIES OF MEDIA CAMPAIGN

Social media portrays different communities with various beliefs. Positive social norms ought to be encouraged and negative ones to be discouraged. Additional motivation can be leveraged through policy changes that support the desired behaviors. Policy enforcement can further discourage unhealthy or unsafe behaviors. Other means of supportive behavioral change come in the form of news and entertainment.

Another challenge is media fracture and clutter environment which is a hindrance to achieving adequate exposure to media messages. Target audience campaign content and format are advised to be carefully planned and tested before being deployed in the campaign process. The difficulty of isolation of independent effects of mass media campaigns does not obstruct the conclusion that mass media campaigns generally prove effective in helping transform healthcare behavior in the targeted society.[93]

More aid is needed by regulators to provide a welcoming ground for interested private sectors in healthcare and media campaign for quick compliance. The state as a regulatory body in charge of registration and regulation of public and private hospitals is expected to examine the processes involved and lighten the burden of investors to encourage their efforts. The Primary Health Centers (SMOH) ought to monitor the health facilities and their registration accordingly. Regulating the healthcare sector is a necessity which is envisioned to be the basic factor in promoting, encouraging, and facilitating Nigerian healthcare. The major requirement for facility registration is the availability of licensed healthcare workers. It is the obligatory function of the Nigerian Nuclear Regulatory Authority (NNRA), a federal agency, to authorize all diagnostic radiography facilities in Nigeria.

Foreign investors in healthcare are also encouraged to participate in establishing hospitals and diagnostic centers in Nigeria following the regulation requirements for foreigners. The same goes to employing expatriates with respect to abiding by the regulatory body policies and laws governing the procedures. This will foster better healthcare, promote well-being, and campaign compliance with positive behaviors. Foreigners bring new medications and new medical ideas to aid, enhance, and influence local officials in healthcare advancement. The need to travel abroad for treatment will be minimal and this will promote savings for citizens as well as the government.

"Businesses that are part of trade missions and bilateral agreements between countries can apply for a waiver for the expatriate quota from the National Planning Commission. Regulating the production and licensing of healthcare workers is the responsibility of federal level councils and boards. Some of the councils also have mandates to inspect and accredit facilities."[94] These are necessary procedures and requirements to be promoted and encouraged by the health sector to improve lives.

INDIRECT INFUSED CAMPAIGNS

Indirect infused campaigns are recommended in some situations and, depending on the community, envisioned to guide behavioral change through exposure to the media. It is a gradual process requiring patience. Media works with the healthcare sector to mobilize the populace on a course that demands practical compliance. Nigerians are health conscious people and are ready to join together in response to media advice on behavioral change. Life is precious and healthcare campaigns involving practical activities that promote living healthy and joining in healthcare programs is valued by Nigerians. It only needs the use of strategic and systematic techniques to produce success.

Most fitness and physical health campaigns are designed with indirect infused campaigns which have proven effective with massive compliance globally. People tend to join gym clubs for physical fitness or dieting clubs for eating right. Suggestions from friends with evidence and reality of their good life belonging to a certain healthcare groups attracts others involved in their social networks. The information circulates from person to person as information is shared and with positive results comes compliance in the society. This works best when a peer group comes together with an idea of how a certain behavior, they wish to either stop or enhance, will benefit them then all they need to do is a set goal on what they want to achieve. Their continuous engagement and pursuit to meet their goals attracts others to either join or start their own efforts. This process keeps involving more people until it becomes the norm or acceptable behavior among people living in that particular community.

FUNDING

The fundamental problem handicapping most media campaigns is lack of sufficient funding. Reaching out to a target community requires constant campaigns to remind people of the necessity of adapting to a new behavior to prevent a certain disease. This is achievable with adequate financing to pay bills on required equipment; wages for health officials; media coverage; insurance if necessary; transportation fares; practical requirements; and more. Government, the stakeholder community, and the private sector can support media campaigns with financing for basic facilities, donations, and others sources of revenue. Funding is a collective effort that demands provision of basic needs for campaigners and media broadcast to ensure information penetration among members of a target audience in a particular community.

"The pattern of health financing is therefore closely and indivisibly linked to the provisioning of services and helps define the outer boundaries of the system's capability to achieve the overall goal of enhancing nation's economic development (Rao, Selvaraju, Nagpal and Sakthivel, 2009). Health care financing therefore does not only involve how to raise sufficient resources to finance health care needs of countries, but also on how to ensure affordability and accessibility of healthcare services, equity in access to medical services as well as guarantee financial risk protection."[95]

Well-funded, long-term campaigns are more effective and are recommended to achieve better results. Communication through media campaigns on healthcare behavioral change for disease prevention demands huge expenditures. Budgets guide every planned campaign must sufficiently fund the activities mapped out at the duration set for the campaign. Unfortunately, without continuous funding on a long-term campaign, most campaigns are destined to fail.

Funding and management are considered to be inseparable for a successful financing of any project. Healthcare leaders and mangers/organizers of campaigns are advised to be transparent and allocate money in the right proportions and places needed, depending on their priority and scale of preference. When money realized from donations, sponsors, stakeholders, and other sources are well-utilized, more funding is likely to flow in the health sector. There will be return on investment for healthcare campaigns resulting in people responding positively to new normal behaviors. Campaigns will be fully deployed and managed constantly throughout the duration of the planned campaign.

PROVISION OF HEALTH CENTERS AND FACILITIES

Provision of health centers and facilities is government's responsibility. The private sector is encouraged to join in national development efforts to help ensure availability and accessibility to healthcare centers and facilities throughout the country. Healthcare centers and facilities ought to be accessible, available, and provide services at a low cost.

It is observed that mass media campaigns can directly or indirectly affect lives and transform individuals or influence large societies to adopt more positive behaviors in the areas of healthcare and health management. From various reviews on how media campaigns work, concurrent availability and access to major services and products are essential tools for persuading individuals and for motivating them, through media messages, to respond to change as directed.

"The fact that the few available facilities are unevenly distributed suggests that health improvement planning in these countries should also pay particular attention to the efficient organization of the available facilities so as to ensure their maximum utilization."[96] Primary Health Care (PHC) centers in Nigeria provide fragmented services, weak referral systems, and poor infrastructure. There are serious gaps to providing easy public access to basic health services. "The multiplicity of vertical disease control programs, with poor integration of services at suboptimal levels, results in low coverage of high-impact, cost-effective interventions. There is poor linkage between the different levels of care. Materials and equipment for service delivery at the PHC facilities are hardly available or functional. Most health centres no longer have functional drug revolving schemes, resulting in shortage of essential and critical medicines and commodities at point of service delivery."[97] Good public health depends upon the ability to ensure that many of the key components of Primary Health Centers are available at service delivery points especially in the rural parts of Nigeria.

REGULATING COMPETING INFLUENCES AFFECTING HEALTHCARE MEDIA CAMPAIGNS

Regulating influences of marketing, usually via advertisements, will help minimize the manipulation of some irresponsible competitions affecting the effectiveness of mass media campaigns on public adherence to a certain behavioral change as expected. Pervasive marketing for competing products or oppositions to media messages, with the power of social norms, and drive of addiction indicates that positive campaign results are not sustainable. This would require greater and long-term investment to extend its effectiveness and achieve compliance.

"Campaigns are often a component of broader social marketing programs. Social marketing is the application of commercial marketing ideas to help solve social and health problems (Andreasen, 1995). Social marketing programs complement communication efforts with other intervention components. For example, a social marketing campaign to encourage childhood vaccination might complement a public communication effort to promote an increase in vaccinations with a subsidy in the price of vaccines and an easier system for obtaining vaccines, or even a change in the rules about what vaccines can be given together.

Aggressive marketing with the recognition of masses heterogeneity, especially in the target audience, is advised to specifically direct unbiased messages without projecting their medical products in the wrong light, thereby influencing the public to buy their products but not confuse the campaign motive. Some campaigns divide their audience into groups according to characteristics of social diversity like age, race, income, gender, or education. It is helpful to direct campaign messages to the proper target audience to minimize expenditure and focus marketing on the target audience. "These are competing criteria for choosing among segments. Once they are understood, the choice among segments is not only a technical decision, but also a political/social/ethical decision. The decision thus may not belong solely in the hands of the project planners, but is appropriately negotiated among the constituencies who have an interest in the outcome." [98]

MULTISECTORIAL AND INTERSECTORAL COLLABORATION

The adoption of multisectoral and intersectoral collaboration by the government to address campaign issues from various spheres is advised to achieve fast and positive outcomes. Encouraging multisectoral and intersectoral collaboration enhance the capacity of engaging cross-bearers of healthcare media campaigns from various fields and sectors. Creating good relationships and trust with open communication promotes a successful campaign.

"The notion that multisectoral and intersectoral collaboration helps to reach the goals of all sectors involved was a key facilitating factor, as was a consensus regarding the action deemed suitable, feasible and acceptable. Additional factors related to the building of strong relationships included effective working methods, quality and reputation of partners and ensuring an appropriate environment to facilitate the receptiveness of different partners to collaborate more broadly." [99] This is achievable by focusing on a clearly identified goals set up to meet the demands of the campaigners.

The motivation drawn from the mutual benefit of a positive result helps strengthen the sectors involved creating a win-win situation. It increases their commitment beyond their boundaries motivating the involvement of other participants in easily adapting to new healthcare behavioral change in the society. "This is crucial in ensuring that nobody is left behind, and nobody falls through gaps in service delivery (e.g. between social, education and health sectors), which is a central element of the 2030 Agenda. More efficient and effective coordination was identified as a mutual benefit that extends beyond health sector. From the health perspective, the benefits of collaboration include an increased capacity to address health challenges, which sometimes includes increased financing for health promoting activities."[100] With the aid of healthcare policies guiding multisectoral and intersectoral collaboration, and the improved method of collaboration, increased coherence will enable more successful campaigns.

"Changes in sectors besides health were reported in 27 of the 36 case stories. The nine cases that did not induce changes in other sectors were limited in their scope, and direct changes across sectors were not necessarily expected. 22 Governance for a sustainable future: improving health and well-being for all. The emphasis on the notion that good health is good for everyone led to the integration of health goals into the activities of non-health sectors. Some of the concrete examples included minimizing the use of antibiotics in livestock (agriculture), reducing the use of salt in food production (agriculture), providing more physical activity and healthier diets in schools (education) and increasing taxes on alcohol and tobacco (finance)."[101]

Some factors facilitated the cooperation of international partners such as the WHO and the EU. The WHO European Healthy Cities Network and the Network of Health Promoting Schools are examples of successful collaborations identified in healthcare which promoted healthcare behaviors involving other sectors outside of the healthcare arena. They effectively disseminated information about problems that require a multisectoral and intersectoral response.[102]

PROPER ENVIRONMENT FOR FITNESS AND PHYSICAL HEALTH PROGRAMS

Provision of a proper environment for fitness and physical health programs is recommended to promote compliance on healthcare behavioral campaigns for physical fitness and wellbeing. Space is very essential in exercising the body. The environment is expected to meet the required standard for extracurricular activities including sports, in some cases. Natural playgrounds and fields used for play ought to be furnished with a recommendable grass. The soil type should be appropriate for human activities. The position and area mapped out for the field should be carefully considered. Some physical activities require an open field while some indoor games need to be well-managed and conducive to indoor spaces. All these and more are handled by the right professionals to protect individuals participating in physical healthcare programs during a workout. A certain standard is expected of physical healthcare givers to measure up in relation to environmental factors before granting them the rights to proceed.

The involvement of physically challenged or handicapped individuals should be provided for and their full-participation accommodated in physical fitness activities, by including paths and walkways designed for wheelchairs. Alternatives to stairs ought to be included for wheelchairs. Schools, hospitals, offices, and other buildings must consider the physically challenged individuals in society as part of the people with the right to access the buildings or physical fitness grounds for a balanced environmental standard in all parts of the country.

Schools are obliged to compulsorily teach physical health subjects and practice exercise to aid media campaigns and government policies on physical health intended to produce positive outcomes. It is recommendable that some schools without standard school play fields, adopt the system of renting recreational spaces during their school's physical exercise and inter-house sports. This effort can be hampered by lack of space and high cost of land in urban areas, especially in Lagos State. Parents are encouraged to bear the children in mind while constructing their family houses to provide space for physical fitness for their children and family members, since exercise benefits everyone.

PRIVATE SECTOR PARTICIPATION IN MEDIA CAMPAIGNS

The private sector is encouraged to participate in media campaigns. When the private healthcare organizations join the government in media campaigns, the health and livelihood of residents improves. The issue of healthcare management demands the participation of everyone. The expected outcome is achieved when some aid is rendered accessing the needs of these private participants in healthcare. "It is important to assess private actors' involvement in the health sector. For example, private actors may not always have the incentives to deal with externalities that affect the availability, accessibility, acceptability, and quality of health care services; they may not be in a position to provide "public goods"; or they may operate under imperfect information."[103]

Most medical officials in Nigeria have the vision to operate hospital, pharmaceutical, midwifery, nursing, physiotherapy and other services to contribute to the well-being and health of the society. They assist the government as copartners in healthcare. Private sector participation entails covering a complex range of activities performed by various types of nongovernmental actors in health sector.[104] The actors are comprised of multi-national corporations, nongovernmental organizations, private institutions as well as charitable bodies and other non-profit entities, and private individuals, such as general practitioners and consultants. Their roles in the delivery of healthcare include health facilities, management of healthcare institutions, manufacturing of healthcare goods and services, and financing of healthcare products and services.

Tracing cases of activities being carried out within a publicly run health care system reveals healthcare support by other organizations or private sector. For instance, in the United Kingdom, private actors in healthcare play their roles in nursing homes for persons with disabilities under the National

Health System. They also participate through public-private partnerships, or in privatized contexts.[105]

RESEARCHERS AND WELL-INFORMED CAMPAIGN PLANNERS

Before embarking on campaigns, campaign planners need to research and strategically provide information in detail. Professionals who design control intervention for outbreak of diseases are epidemiologists, veterinarians, and public health specialists. They depend largely on media in communicating and mobilizing communities through campaigns and publications. This set of professionals are expected to deliver intensive content during campaigns with accurate facts and figures obtained through credible research.

In reference to the COMBI Toolkit by the WHO, it is important to note that the COMBI cannot be successful alone without a structural and strategically planned communication through the campaign planners in conjunction with media functionality. This mobilized the public in accepting the new behavior for a positive change in attacking the infectious Ebola disease. The media disseminating information on the relevance of this toolkit proves how behavioral and social communication interventions can be planned systematically with the right approaches to promote community dialogue with the goal of eradicating such diseases. This is a proactive action needed in surveillance performance of the media campaign planners. Preparation with deep knowledge on the practical aspects of a healthcare campaign is encouraged and necessary to achieve positive results.

Training officials produce outstanding results in media campaigns. Achieving compliance towards a behavioral change requires strategically applied communication through a media campaign. Media sensitization ought to be well-planned with support from the stakeholder-community in training officials to achieve a targeted goal. Multidisciplinary approaches to behavioral change in disease prevention and control are critical to success.

IDENTIFYING THE TARGET AUDIENCE

Every media campaign targets a certain set of individuals in a particular community. It is a crucial fundamental step to trace this group of people and directly involve them in participating in the campaign for it to achieve success. "Medical marketing efforts that attempt to reach anyone, anywhere-are doomed to produce only a squandered budget. Carefully and precisely identifying the target audience is a critical success factor in brand strategy development. You know whom you want to reach, where they are located, what makes them tick [...] and how to speak directly to them."[106]

There are four ways to define the target audience:

- **Geography**: Where are these target audience? What is the actual territory of the campaign plan? This is most times defined by zip codes, within a realistic distance between them and the campaigners' location or locations. (Psychological and physical barriers are considered when dealing with geography).

- **Demographics**: What is the target audience's age, gender, family composition/size, occupation, education, and household income?

- **Psychographics**: What is the general personality, behavior and lifestyle of the target audience? What is their repetition of need? What loyalty characteristics are they like? Are they receptive to new ideas and innovative technology?

- **Behavior**: What are the needs and wants of the target audience? What is their level of knowledge, information sources, consumer patterns or response to the product or service?

When specifically managed and examined, the target audience is best obtained and campaign becomes impactful with expected outcomes.[107]

USE OF TESTIMONIALS FOR ATTRACTIVE CAMPAIGNS

The references regarding the effects of campaigns on the lives of people aid in gaining further target audience attraction. "Social proof is a psychological phenomenon where people conform to the actions of others under the assumption that those actions are reflective of the correct behaviour."[108]

Testimonials serve as a form of review of social proof, convincing people and attracting attention. People verify testimonials to ensure truth is served and when satisfied with their investigations, they tend to refer others to join the trend and the penetration of new behavior is achieved. Testimonials need to be strategically positioned and presented to make impact during healthcare media campaigns. The target audience is presented with its own suitable testimonials depending on the different locations and what type of information seems to be most appealing to members of the audience.

There are some systematic ways of crafting testimonials which include randomly contacting customers to request a testimonial, follow up with recent customers, follow up again later, approach people individually, ask the right questions, and design great testimonials then alongside the testimonial include a name, date, and photograph of the individual who provided it. If possible, include a link to the individual's website for legal proof if one is available.

CHAPTER THREE

Media Coverage of Healthcare Services in the World, Africa, and Nigeria

Overview

Media as a public institution embodies different dimensions in rendering services to humanity. Media operate as an independent entity serving the public. It can be a watchdog probing the activities of the government as a mediating public institution for the people. Media also operates as a private institution with the right to freedom of expression. Media is seen as the fourth estate of the realm. "The derivation of the term Fourth Estate arises from the traditional European concept of the three estates of the realm: the clergy, the nobility, and the commoners.

"Power in most democratic countries is divided between the legislature, executive and judiciary," and "the Fourth Estate keeps government, legislators and big businesses in check by keeping society or the public informed. Investigative journalism plays a big part in uncovering bribery and corruption and in uncovering human rights violations." Google further says that "the term Fourth Estate is commonly used to designate the critical watchdog role of the news media, especially the press, in democratic societies. The expression refers to the concept of the separation of powers, which divides the state into different branches, typically the legislative, executive, and juridical branch."[1]

The media plays a major role in developing other sectors. Harold D. Lasswell, an American political scientist and communications theorist, and Charles R. Wright, professor emeritus of communication and sociology and longtime faculty member of the Annenberg School for Communication at University of Pennsylvania in the US, opined that media is responsible for surveillance of the environment, correlation of parts of society, cultural transmission, and entertainment.[2]

Surveillance of the environment by the media, particularly on healthcare, is the focus of this chapter and has a lot to do with investigative journalism. "An important function of the media is to keep up a surveillance of all the happenings in the world and provide information to the human society. The media has the responsibility of providing news and cover a wide variety of issues that is of some service to the society. Media help maintain social order by providing instructions on what has to be done in times of crisis, thereby reducing confusion among the masses. Example: In times of natural disasters, war, health scares, etc., it is the role of the media to create awareness by providing information on what is happening and of ways in which the disaster can be faced."[3]

The masses have a great dependency on media and their trust on the surveillance responsibility of the media is based on the credibility, accuracy, and reality of the information disseminated by the media. Usually, this trust is obtained from the media organization's past references in serving the public. Despite the challenges facing the contemporary media, media is still seen as the most reliable source for information.

A study by the Media Insight Project, a collaboration of the American Press Institute and the Associated Press-NORC Center for Public Affairs Research, helps establish that trust is an important differentiator for building an audience. The study gathered informative facts with figures on the factors that drive people to trust reporting sources.[4]

The Media Insight Project found that:

- 85% of adults say accuracy is a critical reason they trust a news source
- 76% of adults agree that having the latest details is a critical reason they trust a news source
- 72% of adults value news reporting that's concise and gets to the point
- 63% of digital news consumers believe it is vital ads not interfere
- 79% of political news consumers highly value experts and data in reporting
- 53% of lifestyle news consumers affirm it's important their source is entertaining
- 12% of Facebook news consumers agree that they have lots of trust in the news they access there

It is clear from all indications as stated in the Media Insight Project study conducted in America that media accuracy leads with 85% of adults who believe that accuracy is a critical reason they trust a news source while adults who say having the latest details is a critical reason they trust a news source follows with 76%.

"The study reaffirms that consumers do value broad concepts of trust like fairness, balance, accuracy, and completeness."[5] Since trust is measured with accuracy of information, the media's relevance is attached to its credibility on disseminating accurate information that must be balanced and complete.

"Accuracy is the paramount principle of trust. Eighty-five percent of Americans rate it as extremely or very important that news organizations get the facts right, higher than any other general principle. And when we dig down into more specifics, a particular factor related to accuracy—getting the facts right—is most valued regardless of the topic."[6]

Sourcing information by the media is about verification of the gathered reports. Proof or evidence of the accuracy of the happenings being reported serves as the bedrock on which the audience builds trust and considers the information accurate, and this is the most important factor to be considered by journalists and media institutions. Gaining trust from the audience promotes media and journalist confidence in broadcasting and publishing news content, believing that ears are on the ground listening and eyes are focusing on their ethics. This elevates the professionalism standards of media institutions that processes information the proper way through investigative journalism before publication.

"It has become increasingly important for news media to be trusted. After all, why would people otherwise have more faith in the veracity of information coming from news media compared to that coming from other information sources?" and "why would people otherwise choose to use news media when they can get information from other sources that will provide them with information that confirm their own attitudes and beliefs?"[7]

Media surveillance functionality is an act of fellowship in service for the government, stakeholder communities, and the public. Harold D. Lasswell "identified the surveillance function of the media as instructive in meeting society needs, such as in the process of disease control and prevention."[8]

The job of nearly every media practitioner is seen as a sacrificial service for humanity. Rewards are important to journalists' livelihood and performance, but the best reward is often the satisfaction of a "job well-done" and the impact that was realized from it, especially in the aspect of saving lives through the provision of reliable information. The healthcare sector is a major part of media's responsibility in saving lives and furthering the cause of public health maintenance.

A study conducted in Nigeria "established three points of influence of surveillance campaigns on the society. First is that it could result in negative consequences such as panic if not well managed; it could provide sufficient support for disease management as seen in the Ebola virus disease (EVD) incidence in Nigeria if properly managed; and that effective and well thought-out surveillance campaign will correlate positively in controlling and preventing diseases such as EVD to the point of heightening health education, health promotion and health literacy. All the citizens needed to do is acquire, activate and apply this information to the phenomenon."[9]

The emotional relief of obtaining positive compliance during news updates and campaigns means much to the media. It serves as a measure of the success of their performance and how the information shared with the public penetrated to prove the media competent to the task of positively transforming lives. It is observed that when information is not professionally managed or properly handled, it can lead to a "boomerang effect" which is a situation where the public opts to act upon the opposite of what the media is telling them which would be counterproductive to containment of the relevant disease.

To avoid an unnecessarily negative outcome from the public during information dissemination on disease control, "information managers should ensure strategic management of information on health and diseases."[10] When disease outbreak or other health issues are not well-managed by the media, fear is implanted in the audience and this can skew the essence of the information disseminated. Managing information on health requires strategically skilled media professionals who have experience in fostering stability and calming the public when necessary. Media professionals can and should, when necessary, seek aid from social psychologists who monitor public responses and proffer solutions to situations of disruption in the society.

There are some measures the media has inculcated and positioned to guide its functionality. Gatekeeping is one of them. According to the book *Gatekeeping Theory* by Pamela J. Shoemaker and Time P. Vos, "gatekeeping is one of the media's central roles in public life: people rely on mediators to transform information about billions of events into a manageable number of media messages. This process determines not only which information is selected, but also what the content and nature of messages, such as news, will be. *Gatekeeping Theory* describes the powerful process through which events are covered by the mass media, explaining how and why certain information either passes through gates or is closed off from media attention."[11]

Another definition of gatekeeping states that "gatekeeping is the process of selecting, and then filtering, items of media that can be consumed within the time or space that an individual happens to have. This means gatekeeping falls into a role of surveillance and monitoring data. These gatekeeping decisions are made every day to sort out the relevant items that audiences will see. The gatekeeping theory of mass communication is a method which allows us to keep our sanity. By consuming content that is most relevant to us each day, we can ignore the billions of additional data points that are calling for our attention."[12]

Another review of the book *Gatekeeping Theory* indicates that "gatekeeping is one of the media's central roles in public life: people rely on mediators to transform information about billions of events into a manageable number of media messages. This process determines not only which information is selected, but also what the content and nature of messages, such as news, will be. *Gatekeeping Theory* describes the powerful process through which events are covered by the mass media, explaining how and why certain information either passes through gates or is closed off from media attention."[13]

From the selected definitions of gatekeeping in the media mentioned here, filtration of sources and information surveillance deals with the media monitoring collated data before publishing news for public consumption. There is much reliance on the gatekeepers in the media institution regarding content acceptability.

According to the book *A Primer on Communications Studies*, "gatekeepers function to reinterpret mass media messages. Reinterpretation is useful when gatekeepers translate a message from something too complex or foreign for us to understand into something meaningful. In the lead-up to the Supreme Court's June 2012 ruling on President Obama's health-care-overhaul bill, the media came under scrutiny for not doing a better job of informing the public about the core content and implications of the legislation that had been passed. Given that policy language is difficult for many to understand and that legislation contains many details that may not be important to average people, a concise and lay reinterpretation of the content by the gatekeepers (the media outlets) would have helped the public better understand the bill. Of course, when media outlets reinterpret content to the point that it is untruthful or misleading, they are not ethically fulfilling the gatekeeping function of reinterpretation."[14]

Professionalism in media practices is obtained through education and trainings. There is need for differentiating interpersonal communication from the dissemination of media information to the public. Media professionalism is proven by the characteristics and functions guiding the mass media communication. "One key characteristic of mass communication is its ability to overcome the physical limitations present in face-to-face communication."[15]

The quality of standard media is often measured by how well technology and new media platforms are used. In essence, professionalism in media represents the ability to function with the available technical resources to accomplish a task, accurately, in a timely manner, and while achieving a set goal. "While one person can engage in public speaking and reach one hundred thousand or so people in one of the world's largest stadiums, it would be impossible for one person to reach millions without technology." Additionally, "mass communication draws on fewer sensory channels than face-to-face communication" and "mass media messages involve less interactivity and more delayed feedback than other messages."[16]

Individuals and journalists in the media serve as a type of watchdog on behalf of the public. As a watchdog, the media protects public interests and the government or stakeholders in terms of overall best practices by serving a neutral function on behalf of all stakeholders. "The media can fulfil or fail to fulfill its role as the 'fourth estate' of government—or government 'watchdog.'"[17] This is why the media is seen broadly sourcing content and stabilizing the economic, political, social, scientific, religious, life-saving factors, and more in the society.

A Primer on Communications Studies further explains that "this watchdog role is intended to keep governments from taking too much power from the people and overstepping their bounds. Central to this role is the notion that the press works independently of the government. The 'freedom of the press' as guaranteed by our First-Amendment rights allows the media to act as the eyes and ears of the people. The media is supposed to report information to the public so they can make informed decisions. The media also engages in investigative reporting, which can uncover dangers or corruption that the media can then expose so that the public can demand change."[18] It is quite unfortunate that some media outlets have lost this important attribute.

Expectations of the media in covering news on healthcare is very high and requires resources and specialties in the healthcare sector like medical and pharmaceutical professionals, health workers, stakeholders, government officials, and members of the public to achieve positive outcomes. Healthcare givers render aid in numerous ways. Medication manufacturers (the scientists) provide medicines that prevent and control ailments. Health organizations and the government support the process by implementing healthcare policies, establishing facilities, and more. Compliance from the members of the public based on information consumed from media channels is one way the public can support the media in this endeavor.

Support from the government and stakeholder community is a means for proving the relevance of the media. According to a report entitled The Future of the Public's Health in the 21st Century prepared by the Institute of Medicine (US) Committee on Assuring the Health of the Public in the 21st Century addresses the issues of accessing, managing chronic disease, neglected health care services (i.e., clinical preventive services, oral, and mental health care and substance abuse services), and the capacity of the health care delivery system to better serve the population in terms of cultural competence, quality, functionality, financing, information technology, and emergency preparedness. The study also discusses "the responsibility of the health care system to recognize and play its appropriate role within the inter-sectoral public health system, particularly as it collaborates with the governmental public health agencies."[19]

This study also suggests that "for Americans to enjoy optimal health—as individuals and as a population—they must have the benefit of high-quality health care services that are effectively coordinated within a strong public health system. In considering the role of the health care sector in assuring the nation's health, the committee took as its starting point one of the recommendations of the Institute of Medicine (IOM) report Crossing the Quality Chasm (2001b: 6): "All health care organizations, professional groups, and private and public purchasers should adopt as their explicit purpose to continually reduce the burden of illness, injury, and disability, and to improve the health and functioning of the people of the United States."[20]

The media works in all spheres of life to capture and relay important information related to the security and awareness purposes. This is one of the aspects of the media as a vast industry that requires a significant devotion of manpower. Media's success is driven by its ability to verify news content and valid sources, and provide quick updates in a timely manner in addition to all other activities of the media following standard business procedures with accountability for the results.

Media responsibility on health reports is another means of proving media's importance. The media is obligated to perform their duties responsibly while considering how the public will respond to their reports. "Journalists face unique challenges in covering health news. Some specialized skills, knowledge, and judgment are helpful. For example, some information based on poorly designed or poorly powered studies should not be reported unless the flaws are emphasized. Editors, reporters, and writers need to scrutinize the terminology used in health news. Vague, sensational terms (such as "cure," "miracle," and "breakthrough") may harm news consumers by misleading and misinforming. At the core of journalism's values, such terms should not be used because they are meaningless." [21]

Media institutions investigate their sources and report health information with available links and references, using researchers and private companies, researchers and public institutions, patient advocacy groups and their sponsors, celebrity spokespersons and their sponsors, and non-profit health and professional organizations and their sponsors. Making good use of these available resources contributes to the goal of media reports being unbiased and balanced in the reporting of health information.

Basic Roles of Healthcare Journalists and Problems Identified

INFORM AND EDUCATE THE PUBLIC ON HEALTHCARE AWARENESS AND THE ENVIRONMENT

One of the major roles of healthcare journalists is to inform and educate people on health awareness and happenings around them regarding any current health crisis. "Health journalists can communicate to inform and educate people about ways to enhance healthy living in all sorts of countries – developed, developing or undeveloped; besides, they are powerful enough to encourage a people-friendly health policy and/or health communication strategy through many a measures such as: increase the level of knowledge and awareness of a health issue among a certain audience influence and/or change behaviours and attitudes towards a health issue, educate healthy practices, demonstrate the benefits of behaviour changes to public health outcomes."[22]

Focusing on informing and educating the public means healthcare journalists must provide credible health updates and even distribution of healthcare information to promote healthy living in various communities around the world. According to an article published in PLOS MEDICINE regarding the roles and responsibilities of the media in disseminating health information, "some journalists say that their role and responsibility is no different in covering health information than it is in covering politics, business, or any other topic. These journalists say that their primary concern is accurate, clear reporting—they are less concerned about the consequences of their story once it is published. But that approach may result in shoddy journalism and potential harm to the public. I assert that it isn't sufficient to be accurate and clear when covering health news. Journalists have a responsibility to mirror a society's needs and issues, comprehensively and proportionally. Often that doesn't happen in health news."[23]

Journalism in healthcare is dimensional in sourcing information regarding health, determinants of health and medical services. The masses need to first be aware of the disease or health issue they are to prevent or control, before updates on medications saturates the media, causing confusion on what is more important. "Journalists must weigh the balance between the amount of attention given to news about medicine and the attention given to news about health and the social determinants of health. There may be too much news about the delivery of medical services and not enough news about the cost of, quality of, and evidence for those services."[24] When journalists support contents on promotions of medical companies marketing their products over important healthcare information, brands of available medications start occupying the entire media spectrum. The focus becomes medications seeking customers and vital healthcare measures for preventing the health crisis or disease information which are more essential for public health are not adequately communicated to the public.

POLICY AND SOCIAL INFLUENCERS ON HEALTH ISSUES

Professional healthcare journalists lead by practicing what they preach. Journalists are not only encouragers of good health practices while being proactive on good measures for healthy living, but they demonstrate their civic duty by influencing others. They encourage health leaders to take available vaccines they promote to provide proof to convince the public, especially those that may have doubts, with regard to the safety of the medications. "Increase demand and support for health services help the concerned authorities understand the necessity of increased numbers of platforms (i.e., websites, software/apps) to be initiated, and increase access to them, increase ethical and responsible reporting on healthcare issues widely covering issues regarding best and accurate use of medicines.

Keeping the society aware of issues regarding the broad context of medicine use, risks of medicine use, non-drug alternatives etc. Diminish misconceptions about different health issues, and above all advocate a position on a health issue or policy/strategy."[25]

In cases of casualties in connection with new medications, it is the responsibility of health journalists to write reports and minimize the use of the medication through press releases and publications. Health is about life and death and so must be addressed as quickly as possible when negative observation or occurrences arise. It does not matter the source of the medications or who manufactured them; what matters is saving lives, and journalists are expected to investigate the impact and reactions to new medications before encouraging the public to employ them. For instance, the recent COVID-19 vaccine has a lot of myths surrounding it and this poses a challenge to healthcare journalists in convincing the public to accept it. This is why investigation is very necessary to prove or disprove public rumors and myths with actual proof.

According to the WHO Regional Office for Africa, "supporting media to bust harmful myths on coronavirus disease by WHO held in Abuja, 13 February 2020 states, that "From eating garlic to gargling with mouthwash, the public space is full of information about how to prevent coronavirus disease. However, much of this is misinformation. To counter this spread of harmful rumours, the World Health Organization (WHO) is organizing workshops in many African countries to inform media professionals on the facts about COVID-19."[26]

"For Dhamari Naidoo, the WHO emergency officer who conducted the training, 'journalists and media are critical to getting the right messages to the community.' She urged them to ensure that accurate information was shared with the public and reminded reporters of the key role they play in preventing the spread of fake news: 'There is a need for journalists to be precise and concise when sharing information to citizens. We want you to transmit the right information to the people, and to contribute in stopping the spread of rumors.'"[27]

Journalists working under the health sector are encouraged to take an active role in healthcare workshops organized by a valid stakeholder in healthcare such as WHO to keep the pace in strategizing how to combat myths and misinformation surrounding good medical practices by world standard health organizations for disease containment. "Maliki Duro, a correspondent with Airview news said: 'This is really an eye opener. The orientation will avail Nigerian journalists with first-hand information as well as enhance their capacity to accurately report information related to the outbreak.'"[28] A journalist testifies during an interview about the workshop that "there has been a lot of misinformation about the novel coronavirus out there. This workshop has empowered me with knowledge. I can now differentiate between true and false information', said Godsgift Onyedinefu, a reporter with Business Day Newspapers in Abuja. Onyedinefu was one of 54 journalists who participated in a recent workshop, which took place in Abuja, Nigeria."[29]

HEALTH INFORMATION AND CAMPAIGN PROMOTION THROUGH OTHER DEPARTMENTS UNDER MEDIA

Journalists are expected to reach out to other sectors involving healthcare communication for fast penetration of information in the system and to achieve a quick positive response using their media departments. "Healthcare is a continuum of structures and principles enshrined in a normative and operative framework aiming to interact in harmony, and attainment of which hinges on the mutual adaptation with other areas of the knowledge economy. Developing a knowledge-based economic system by leveraging social capital and underpinning research and organizational culture holds great promises to overcome the most pertinent organizational and communication issues on global health."[30]

Integrating health information in entertainment media, social media marketing, interpersonal communication, media-mix approach (e.g. interpersonal, group, organizational, and mass media), and more enhances media reach in different segments and communities. It is a good strategy for communicating healthcare covering numerous regions to achieve positive results among members of different organizations as well as rural habitants. The aid of new technology has improved health information outreach in remote areas as healthcare journalists partner with telecommunication companies in the delivery of health information providing remote accessibility through the use of mobile phones and other electronic devices. This helps improve the quality of life across all sectors of society.

According to *mHealth New horizons for health through mobile technologies, a* report published by the WHO, "the unprecedented spread of mobile technologies as well as advancements in their innovative application to address health priorities has evolved into a new field of eHealth, known as mHealth. According to the International Telecommunication Union, there are now close to five billion mobile phone subscriptions in the world, with over 85% of the world's population now covered by a commercial wireless signal. The penetration of mobile phone networks in many low- and middle-income countries surpasses other infrastructure such as paved roads and electricity, and dwarfs fixed internet deployment. The growing sophistication of these networks – offering higher and higher speeds of data transmission alongside cheaper and more powerful handsets – are transforming the way health services and information are accessed, delivered, and managed. With increased accessibility comes the possibility of greater personalization and citizen-focused public health and medical care."[31]

By definition "mHealth is a component of eHealth. To date, no standardized definition of mHealth has been established."[32] The report continues, "Global Observatory for eHealth (GOe) defined mHealth or mobile health as medical and public health practice supported by mobile devices, such as mobile phones, patient monitoring devices, personal digital assistants (PDAs), and other wireless devices." This strategy will encompass other sectors faster and easily since its means of accessibility can cut across with phones owned by majority of world's population irrespective of location. It is interesting that government has shown interest in mHealth. "Governments are expressing interest in mHealth as a complementary strategy for strengthening health systems and achieving the health-related Millennium Development Goals (MDGs) in low- and middle-income countries."[33]

IDENTIFYING THE KEY STAKEHOLDERS IN HEALTHCARE AND ESTABLISHING A PROFESSIONAL RELATIONSHIP

Healthcare journalists, as professionals, need to observe their working environment and consider the functionality of their stakeholder community as a component of their success. This will help in aligning them to the requirements for the necessary processes involved in sourcing health information and reports. "Specific stakeholders can be identified from the following sectors: international/donors, national political (legislators, governors), public (Ministry of Health [MOH], social security agency, ministry of finance), labor (unions, medical associations), commercial/private for-profit, and nonprofit (nongovernmental organizations [NGOs], foundations). Civil society is an important sector to consider if the community or consumers have a direct interest in the policy. It is also important to consider the potential stakeholders in different geographic or administrative areas within one organization."[34]

"More in-depth engagement of cross-professional stakeholders is desirable to ensure best practice and harnessing the benefits of collective approach. Mutual collaboration for wealth and knowledge creation and management within the healthcare industry can be greatly facilitated by the active involvement of health journalism which is still a largely unexplored domain in the context of developing countries. In addition, health journalism has a lot to contribute in bridging the gap between global north and south in terms of cooperation in healthcare research and exchange of information and expertise which are fundamental to the advancement of knowledge economy."[35]

In identifying the stakeholder community within the health sector for journalists, the following steps are recommended by the WHO in the publication *Stakeholder Analysis Guidelines, Section 2* authored by Kammi Schmeer.[36]

- **Identifying the key stakeholders** is extremely important to the success of the analysis. Based on the resources available, the working group should decide on the maximum number of stakeholders to be interviewed. The working group should then follow the steps below to define the list of stakeholders (beginning with an open list that can be reduced, if necessary).

- **Compile and review existing information**, the working group should gather and analyze any written documents related to the selected policy. This will help to identify potential stakeholders and, perhaps, their connection to the policy.

- **Develop a list of all possible stakeholders**, Initially, the working group should identify all actors who could have an interest in the selected policy, including actors outside the health sector that could affect or be affected by the policy.

- **Develop a list of priority stakeholders** with input from experts. Since resources, time, and finances for the analysis will be limited, the list of stakeholders to be interviewed must be prioritized. Experts who know the sector, policy, and players can help in this process."

Best practices in terms of the recommended steps for journalists deals with segmentation of working groups depending on the stakeholders for which they are responsible. "The working group should consult with two to three persons who have extensive knowledge of the health sector, its actors, and the power of those actors to influence the policy. Experts could be representatives from donor organizations, health reform projects, a national health council, private consulting firms that have worked in health, or other sector-wide organizations. They could also be persons who have worked in various positions in the health sector, such as ex-MOH authorities. Ideally, these experts should not be stakeholders themselves. Two working group members should meet with the experts to identify potential stakeholders from the various sectors. The discussion should focus on persons or organizations that may be related to or affected by the particular policy and that have the ability to affect the implementation of the policy."[37]

UNDERSTANDING THE COMPLEXITY OF HEALTHCARE SYSTEM AND IMPROVING TRANSFORMATIONAL METHODOLOGIES

The healthcare sector is a complex sphere requiring journalists to be guided and recognize its complexity to enable them understand how health professionals work with them. "Understanding healthcare delivery as a complex adaptive system will help us design a system that yields better health outcomes."[38] This same study provides "possible benefits from a range of technologies, including electronic health records and telemedicine; data mining as an alternative to randomized trials; conceptual and analytical methodologies that address the complexity of the healthcare system; and how these principles, models, and methods can enable transformational change."[39]

"An awareness of how to work with the media is essential for health communicators. This includes understanding journalists' daily routines, being available, providing resources, and building relationships with specialist health reporters." The result of the study proves that "Journalists routinely attempted to balance different, sometimes competing, aims amidst significant operational constraints. They perceived the most trusted sources on health issues to be respected and independent doctors. Specialist health and medical reporters had a more sounding technical knowledge, channels to appropriate sources, power within their organizations, and ability to advocate for better quality coverage."[40]

Healthcare journalists should not let their differences by nature or job specifications reduce their productivity or impact their ability to deliver quality work. Experienced journalists ought to train and encourage new journalists to fill their space when they retire or withdraw from the profession. "The fact that health professionals and journalists have different values and goals – not to mention different concepts of validity, objectivity and significance – is as well-known as the frustrations that arise from these differences. Journalists tend to use anecdotal or rhetorical rather than statistical evidence; rely on expert testimony rather than on publications; emphasize controversy rather than consensus; and represent issues in terms of polarities rather than complexities. There are significant barriers to increasing quality of health and medical reporting. These include: lack of technical training for journalists, the time constraints of news production, and the commercial imperatives that drive story selection and headlines."[41]

CAPACITY BUILDING BY EMPOWERING NEW HEALTHCARE JOURNALISTS

Empowering others within the organization is an essential component for the preservation of healthcare journalism. Some experts hoard knowledge forgetting they were empowered by others to serve the public interest. Journalists must further the transfer of knowledge to sustain the system. In-house training conferences and workshops create avenues for new journalists to ask questions and gain knowledge in the field of journalism. Training in the office and during field work with regard to time management is also recommended.

Some of the frustrations that arise among journalists is fear of losing their jobs and being replaced with better employees. This sometimes results in older journalists being apprehensive about imparting knowledge to the younger ones, thereby hindering growth and advancement. New journalists are expected to be curious and work hard in learning and acquiring more skills from the older employees as well. Collaboration at work in sourcing information from stakeholder community has to include a process of replenishment to empower a new generation of journalists in the knowledge and practices involved in the various stages of news reporting. Experience goes a long way in preparing new participants as part of the system.

The Inter Press Service (IPS) is one of the capacity building processes which empowers journalists and offers a platform designed to enhance journalists' ability to perform as experts. "IPS training experiences are intended to hone the professional skills of participants, deepen their knowledge and networks and to contribute to transformational change by providing new frames of reference. Training is seen not just as an event but as a process, so IPS trainings encompass customized preparation by the trainers, the physical event and follow-up.

"As part of many of its larger training programs IPS prepares and distributes training manual, tools and guidelines on important development issues for journalists, media houses and experts. IPS is keen to move from static online training resources to a more interactive offering.

"IPS training capacity is situated alongside the work of the IPS daily news agency, ensuring that the training is grounded and immediately relevant to or connected with working journalists. On occasion the trainees have the opportunity to pitch [their employability attainments] to editors in the news agency during and after their training experience."[42]

"Building internal communications capacity means providing timely and effective information to all staff, connecting offices across the organization, and promoting stronger employee engagement; corporate priority events, such as global public health days, facilitating dialogue and information exchange are prime avenues. The headquarters team also manages the corporate intranet homepage: ensuring it contains critical, up-to-date information for staff about programme, management, and staff initiatives, and regular features on individual staff members from around the world."[43]

The *WHO Strategic Communications Framework for effective communications*, a publication by the WHO, recommends that communicators and journalists "should consider these questions when designing communications actions and products that are timely. When health threats are urgent, what are the best methods to engage priority audiences quickly? When are the audiences likely to be faced with a health-related decision for themselves or others on the health topic? How can messages be delivered so that audiences have enough time to understand and act on the message? How can WHO best engage with the press to get messages to the public quickly? Are there times when a health message will be crowded out by competing issues and concerns? Is there a way to deliver a sequence of messages over time that would increase the effectiveness of information and advice? How can WHO support partners so there is timely and consistent dissemination of information and advice?"[44]

ATTENDING HEALTH CONFERENCES AND COORDINATING HEALTHCARE CAMPAIGNS

Journalists need to create and monitor more healthcare programs involving key stakeholders in health and other sectors. During global or regional conferences, when dignitaries and reputable professionals in healthcare services are present, journalists are expected to conduct interviews and disseminate information to the public. Healthcare journalists can coordinate public health campaigns with available professionals to facilitate effective interaction between the public and the doctors, ministry of health personalities, WHO members, and more in attendance at such events.

"In order for healthcare service industry in emerging economies stay competitive in today's complex and volatile economic environment, understanding the interest of different stakeholders, and how their influence shape various domains of social development is crucial. The magnitude of the task is overwhelming and success will depend on integrative approach by local and international actors in strategic decision making and translating to concrete policy framework which will provide the key for long term success for healthcare institutions' key messages regarding the necessity of cross-professional communication in health sector development are stated in the study, proving the essentiality of collaborating with health professionals from different fields and backgrounds during intra and international gatherings for tackling issues on healthcare. The study also states that healthcare professionals' communication with journalists is part of "the role of health journalism as a potential instrument for strengthening health policy advocacy, developing international standards in communication and more effective knowledge management."[45]

Important reasons for healthcare journalists to be encouraged in attending conferences and healthcare programs are numerous. As communicated in the article "Medical Conferences: 'Should I Stay or Should I Go?'"

appearing in *Health eCareers*, a survey from Ogilvy Health Worldwide found out that the reasons for attending healthcare conferences and other programs are as follows: Learn about new clinical information. Keep with current trends. Get continuing medical education (CME). Participate in professional networking. Collect material for personal knowledge. Meet with specific company representatives. Enjoy entertainment.[46]

Testimonies of attendees at healthcare conferences were also reported in the article. "'I attend two or three medical conferences per year, and I find them to be very beneficial,' says Sylvia Stacy, M.D., M.P.H. 'The main reasons are networking with others in the same field and keeping up to date on trends, advances and hot topics in the field. I'm an introvert, and I have to push myself to get out there and take advantage of everything that most conferences offer, such as sessions, roundtables, exhibit halls, mixers and workshops, but I never regret it when I participate in this stuff. I always take away a new relationship, a new piece of knowledge, a new professional goal or an idea to dwell on.' A chief medical officer, Richard Honaker, M.D. shares a rousing, 'Go!' He says, 'I love medical conferences. To remain board certified, I need 50 hours of education every year. If I do not attend conferences, I feel really out of date.' Pulmonary and critical-care physician Sachin Gupta, M.D. states, "Medical conferences come in a variety of styles and formats. As a subspecialist in pulmonary hypertension, I attend conferences related to this disease state as a means of learning about the latest in research, innovation and therapies."[47]

Recommendations

These recommendations serve as processes to be recognized in correcting issues in connection to basic roles of healthcare journalists and problems identified.

INVESTIGATIVE JOURNALISM TO BE MONITORED IN HEALTHCARE

More is expected of the media as a public institution. The media must work hard to maintain a high level of trust with their audience. This is only possible when investigations produce accurate facts and figures that are reported to the public. "In some cases, investigative reporters have exposed aspects of medicine and medical science that prompted legislative and policy changes in the health care system. For example, a New York Times probe of fraudulent practices at the Columbia/HCA Healthcare Corp chain of hospitals in March 1997 led to a federal criminal investigation of the company. A Los Angeles Times series on the US Food and Drug Administration's system of drug approval in 2000 strengthened the claims of those advocating tighter controls at the agency. Extensive coverage by the Washington Post and others of the death of a young patient in a university-based gene therapy experiment resulted in stronger federal protections for patients enrolled in clinical trials. A Boston Globe series on the hazards of placebo-controlled trials in psychiatry was one of several journalistic investigations that resulted in changes in the way psychiatric patients are enrolled in research protocols."[48]

News content and the verification of sources with existing references need thorough examination before journalists arrive and report a definite conclusion. If not properly investigated, reporting could have unexpected results on society. Most times, this is in connection with new medications (vaccines). Reporters need to be familiar with basic scientific knowledge to aid their overall ability in investigating medical reports accurately.

"Physicians and scientists have criticized journalists for misleading the public about important medical issues. For example, a 1997 survey of scientists found that the majority of them believed that reporters do not understand statistics well enough to explain new scientific findings, do not understand the nature of science and technology, and are more interested in sensationalism than in scientific truth. These concerns may have been bolstered by misleading reports in the popular press. For instance, sensationalized reports on the hazards of calcium channel blockers may have led some patients to stop taking their prescribed antihypertensive medications, while optimistic coverage of rodent experiments in the field of antiangiogenesis resulted in patients with cancer requesting this unproven treatment from their oncologists."[49] This is when investigative journalism goes wrong. Healthcare journalists must be vigilant in avoiding such outcomes from their reporting.

STRATEGIC PLANS BY THE MEDIA ARE NEEDED FOR STAGE-MANAGING NEGATIVE RESPONSES ON HEALTH REPORTS

Situation assessment involves risk management as well as emergency management with proper strategic response in handling negative responses to health-related reporting. According to a report on responding to the Novel Coronavirus published in 2019 by the WHO, "the Emergency Committee also provided advice to the WHO, and welcomed a forthcoming WHO-led multidisciplinary and multi-partner technical mission to China. The mission will review and support efforts to investigate the animal source of the outbreak, the clinical spectrum of the disease and its severity, the extent of human-to-human transmission in the community and in healthcare facilities, and efforts to control the outbreak. This mission will provide information to the international community to aid in understanding the situation, its impact, and effective public health measures to respond to the virus."[50] This is one of the strategic ways of controlling negative responses from the audience in managing situational health crisis.

Additional strategic ways of managing reporting in times of crisis require "rapidly establishing international coordination to deliver strategic, technical, and operational support through existing mechanisms and partnerships, scaling up country preparedness and response operations, including strengthening readiness to rapidly identify, diagnose and treat cases; identification and follow-up of contacts when feasible (with priority given to high-risk settings), [...] awareness raising in the population through risk communication and community engagement, and accelerating priority research and innovation to support a clear and transparent global process to set research and innovation priorities to fast track and scale-up research, development [...] This will build a common platform for standardized processes, protocols and tools, to facilitate multidisciplinary and collaborative research integrated with the response."[51]

Tackling problematic media reporting must consider the local, regional, national, and global level entities impacted by the crisis to ensure effective coordination of international partners and the stakeholders involved. Teams of journalists need to be deployed to cut across different geographical levels. "These teams ensure regular communication between incident managers at different geographical levels of the response, and close operational coordination with national governments, partners across all sectors, and services at all levels."[52] This guidance from the UN Inter-Agency Standing Committee (IASC) and the WHO targeting operators at the global and local levels. Journalists are advised to set up a monitoring framework and follow up on the measures taken by these reputable international organizations in forecasting, coordinating, and managing cases by seeking aid when necessary to disseminate accurate and existing evidence.

ALL MEDIA ACTIVITIES TO FOLLOW MEDIA PROCEDURES AND BE ACCOUNTABLE

In consideration of quick and timely updates, it is recommended that activities of the media including sourcing data, collation of data, writing and editing of news reports, publishing, and all media practices ought to be guided by existing protocols. This will enhance productivity and accuracy with proper levels of screening to ensure standard finished products of the media publications.

Nonproductive attitudes at work should be addressed with accountability to resolve the issue. Older journalists should lead capable individuals in proper media practices. The fear of losing jobs should be less of a problem when journalists upgrade their skills. Promotions can serve as a competitive strategy of enforcing and rewarding positive attitudes. The recent unemployment issue has contributed to this. There is need for more job creation to eliminate the unnecessary fear of journalists losing their jobs to new staff. It should be resolved with media expansion. The advantage of media as a broad area, yet to be taped in most aspects of journalism, should be configured to produce more opportunities to strengthen job security.

GATEKEEPING IN MEDIA NEEDS ACTIVATION AND IMPROVEMENT

A thesis written in 2013 and entitled *The Relevance of Gatekeeping the Process of Contemporary News Creation and Circulation in Saudi Arabia* by Abdullah Almaghlooth, a student at the University of Salford School of Arts and Media reported that gatekeeping themes emerged from the observations of the research and it serves as a guide for gatekeeping techniques using systematic operations with division of labor among gatekeepers.[53] The themes are as follows:

- Communication routines

- Social gatekeeping and women's issues
- Governmental gatekeeping
- Audience gatekeeping
- Religious gatekeeping
- Personal attitudes
- Hard versus soft-copy gatekeeping
- Blocking
- Post-production gatekeeping

The model used in gatekeeping depends on the contents sourced and should be guided by proper media standards of publishing reports, considering that influence of any sort is not acceptable on cases treated while gatekeeping. "Shoemaker and Reese (1996) argue that the factors affecting the decisions of gatekeepers include news values, government, culture, personal judgment, politics, ethics, and beliefs."[54] Health publications should not be biased or controlled by a single person or an institution. Gatekeepers should resolve such issues before news reports are publicized.

"Journalists (gate-keepers) should be systematic by the processes involved in gate-keeping in segmentations to quickly identify some irrelevant or disrupting contents that are not qualified to be published. The scrutinizing or screening stages need more examinations and thorough checks. The media should involve strict measures in gate-keeping by examining how gatekeeping is currently applied to health news content [...], with regard to print newspapers, e-newspapers, blogs and Twitter microblogs. The prevalence of the internet means that the creation and circulation of news are undergoing dramatic changes, which in turn affect the operation of gatekeeping and the processing of news. This has to be checked with measures by blocking the contents using technology.

"The media need to identify the new gatekeepers emerging in the health media landscape, due to the development of various technologies and health information on disease outbreaks, which impact the creation and circulation of news. Their qualifications for publication should be investigated and disqualified if not satisfactorily acceptable as standard media content. Journalists are advised to improve gatekeeping theory in order to accommodate the changes occurring in the digital age."[55]

POSITIONING OF MEDIA INSTITUTIONS AS WATCHDOGS AND FOURTH ESTATE OF THE REALM ON HEALTH CASES

"When the media releases information to motivate or inspire the public or rather the Nigerian citizenry towards a particular set agenda, it is performing its role as a fourth estate of the realm. For example, carrying out campaigns on health issues such as HIV/AIDS, Polio, Cholera, and the Ebola virus motivates the public to take extra precautions on their health."[56] Initiation of more healthcare campaigns and conferences to motivate and inspire the public on health matters is highly needed, especially in the current situation with the COVID-19 pandemic and other disturbing diseases and infections.

The role of the media as the fourth estate of the realm should embody the watchdog functionality in defending the public's right to know by promoting freedom of the press in tackling healthcare issues. For instance, the new vaccine for COVID-19 is out. The media should investigate and follow up on the vaccine producers to verify that they are first in-line in adhering to compliance on being vaccinated for proof of safety before urging citizens to comply.

The media is a fearless institution that the public depends upon for lifesaving guidance at a time when so many are exposed to dangers. Media disclosure of leaders' unworthy activities motivates the public in demanding government accountability. According to the article, *Role of Media during the COVID-19 Pandemic & its Impact on Medication* authored by Monalisa Changkija, "these pandemic times demand that we need to keep a sharper eye right from civil and human rights protection or violations of our health workers and other front-liners, women, children, disabled, the elderly, minorities and other vulnerable sections, etc., to policy making that inevitably impact on every section of society and paves the way for our future one way or the other. If we lose sight of, and let our guard down from, constitutional provisions and the imperatives of transparency and accountability of those in power, we will fail in our role as the watchdog of society and negate the very reasons for our existence."[57]

Journalists are encouraged to keep an eye as the watchdogs in service to humanity at this critical time of Corona virus pandemic to justify their honorable position as the fourth estate of the realm.

INTEGRATION OF HEALTHCARE COMMUNICATION ACROSS ALL SECTORS BY ENCOURAGING THE NEW INITIATIVES EHEALTH AND MHEALTH

Using mobile phones in accessing healthcare information is relatively new and should be encouraged. "A prime reason for the growing popularity and awareness of eHealth is the advancement in computer and communication technology which has made the healthcare information and services globally accessible at a very low cost. According to Dr. T. E. Bell (IEEE spectrum 2006) the effective and efficient use of engineering can lower the costs provided. it is focused on early detection of the disease. Different factors are participating in driving towards a better implementation and wider use of eHealth services and technologies."[58]

The role of four important technologies, namely, satellite, internet, mobile, and cloud for providing health services has to be infused among journalists' as essential resourceful skills needed for blending with the new strategy of serving the populace. A few advantages of eHealth technologies are listed in the following:[59]

- With the advent of new and modern technologies, voice and data in form of pictures, videos, and text can be relayed in real time on various types of computing devices, even mobile handsets.

- Multi-location real time videoconference can be used to conduct training sessions, live demonstrations, collaborations, and so forth.

- Simple internet connection can be used by large number of people to study and to gain knowledge about health-related issues at their own convenience.

- eHealth services may play an important role in maintaining the doctor-patient ratio all round the world.

- Electronic health records (EHR) of the patients may be maintained which in turn may be beneficial to the medical practitioners in treatment of diseases.

- Providing medical facility to elderly is the most challenging task in today's world. The World Health Organization has estimated that the proportion of persons over 60 years of age will double to 22% in 2050 from 11% in 2000. Thus, over two billion people will require additional medical support, even assisted living, as they will be more prone to health-related issues. The aging society can be served by satellite based medical diagnosis and care from their homes.

mHealth (or mobile health) is "an emerging innovation that capitalizes on the features and ubiquity of mobile phones across the globe to facilitate communication between patients and health institutions, to deliver health services, and to promote health preventive behaviors (Pattichis, Istepanian,

& Laxminarayan, 2006, p. 3)."[60] Importance of mHealth is immeasurable and it has proven to be very successful as claimed by the study.

"The articulation of mHealth as instrumental to generating positive health outcomes in communities across Asia erases the contexts within which mobile technologies are constituted. mHealth interventions reproduce the logics of the state and the market, reproducing communities as homogeneous and monolithic sites of top-down interventions."[61] The situation of a woman in labor in a remote location describes the role of mHealth played when an ordinary person was able to lend a valuable hand without any knowledge of midwifery. The assistance of the untrained midwife with the aid of mobile communications on mHealth successfully saved the life of the mother and child.

Healthcare is made easier, faster, and accessible within seconds at any location and any time through mHealth. With mHealth, the number of clinical visits by patients are said to have drastically reduced. "The World Health Organization's global survey (WHO, 2011) reveals a range of uses of mobile technologies in health communications. Such technologies are being used to improve (1) communication from patient to health service providers (e.g., health hotlines or call centers); (2) communication from health service providers to patients (e.g., SMS reminders for appointments, compliance with treatments, or information to raise awareness); (3) health consultations over the mobile phone; (4) communication among health services in emergencies; (5) monitoring and surveillance of patient's health; and (6) the accessibility of databases of patient records (World Health Organization, 2011)."[62]

ABOUT THE AUTHOR

Mary-Jane Ilozor is an author, speaker, communications expert, TV producer, and freelance journalist. She owns and operates Digital Alliance Ltd., a leading ICT systems integration company which she founded in 2010 focusing on delivery of enterprise ICT solutions, cyber security and services, and creative content to small, medium, and large-scale businesses in Nigeria and Africa.

She obtained her first degree in English Language and Literature at Nnamdi Azikiwe University (UNIZIK) and also earned master's degrees in English Literature from University of Lagos as well as in Media and Communications from Pan-Atlantic University. Her study of English literature covered classic essays by Plato and Aristotle to medieval classics of Shakespeare to the modern writings of Martin Luther King, Jr. and Maya Angelo, as well as the contemporary works of Chinua Achebe, Emecheta, Wole Soyinka, J.P. Clarks, Chimamanda Adichie and others.

She highlights her passion for elevating public health and well-being by having focused one of her master's case studies on the link between public health and timely, accurate media communications. The findings of that research serve as the basis for her first book, *Influence of Media on Public Health: Solutions to Healthcare Surveillance Issues in Nigeria, Africa and Around the World.*

As an experienced information and communications technology (ICT) sales professional with over six years of experience in the industry and over nine years of experience as a communications expert, Mary-Jane Ilozor is a talented writer/researcher with a consultative and methodical approach towards achieving results. Her professional growth is motivated by a focused and holistic approach to improving business value and performance backed by her wealth of business acumen and continuing educational journey.

GLOSSARY

CME   continuing medical education

COMBI   Communication for Behavioral Impact

CVD   cardiovascular disease

CBE   clinical breast exam

DCBE   double contrast barium enema

EHR   electronic health records

EVD   Ebola virus disease

FCTC   Framework Convention on Tobacco Control

FMOH   Federal Ministry of Health

FOBT   fecal occult blood test

GOe   Global Observatory for eHealth

IASC   Inter-Agency Standing Committee

ICT   information and communications technologies

IOM	Institute of Medicine
IPS	Inter Press Service
MDG	Millennium Development Goals
MOH	Ministry of Health
NGO	nongovernmental organization
NIH	National Institute of Health
NNRA	Nigerian Nuclear Regulatory Authority
NPHCDA	National Primary Health Care Development Agency
PDA	personal digital assistant
PHC	Primary Health Care
SMOH	Primary Health Centers
UN	United Nations
US	United States
USA	United States of America
WHO	World Health Organization

REFERENCES

Introduction

[1] Omipidan, Teslim. (2016, March 30). Iwe Irohin – The First Newspaper in Nigeria. *OldNaija*. https://oldnaija.com/2016/03/30/iwe-irohin-the-first-newspaper-in-nigeria

[2] A brief walk into the origin of local print media. (2018, February 6). *Pulse.ng*. https://www.pulse.ng/news/local/history-of-nigerian-newspaper-a-brief-walk-into-the-origin-of-local-print-media/d7yqm4d

[3] A brief walk into the origin of local print media. (2018, February 6). *Pulse.ng*. https://www.pulse.ng/news/local/history-of-nigerian-newspaper-a-brief-walk-into-the-origin-of-local-print-media/d7yqm4d

[4] *The Story of Africa Between World Wars (1914-1945)*. BBC World Service. http://www.bbc.co.uk/worldservice/africa/features/storyofafrica/13chapter7.shtml#

[5] A brief walk into the origin of local print media. (2018, February 6). *Pulse.ng*. https://www.pulse.ng/news/local/history-of-nigerian-newspaper-a-brief-walk-into-the-origin-of-local-print-media/d7yqm4d

[6] A brief walk into the origin of local print media. (2018, February 6). *Pulse.ng*. https://www.pulse.ng/news/local/history-of-nigerian-newspaper-a-brief-walk-into-the-origin-of-local-print-media/d7yqm4d

[7] *The Story of Africa Between World Wars (1914-1945)*. BBC World Service. http://www.bbc.co.uk/worldservice/africa/features/storyofafrica/13chapter7.shtml#

[8] *A brief walk into the origin of local print media*. (2018, February 6). Pulse.ng. https://www.pulse.ng/news/local/history-of-nigerian-newspaper-a-brief-walk-into-the-origin-of-local-print-media/d7yqm4d

[9] *About Us*. Nigerian Tribune. https://tribuneonlineng.com/about-us

[10] *List of Nigerian magazines and journals*. W3newspapers. https://www.w3newspapers.com/nigeria/magazines

[11] Overview print media. Oxford Reference. https://www.oxfordreference.com/view/10.1093/oi/authority.20110803100346392

[12] Maringues, Michèle. (2001). The Nigerian Press: Current state, travails and prospects. *OpenEdition Books*. https://books.openedition.org/ifra/640?lang=en

Chapter One

[1] Overview print media. Oxford Reference. https://www.oxfordreference.com/view/10.1093/oi/authority.20110803100346392

[2] Otana, Okinm-Alobi.Okpara, Ngozi. (2017, October). *Health Communication: The Responsibility of the Media in Nigeria*. ResearchGate. https://www.researchgate.net/publication/320265191_Health_Communication_The_Responsibility_of_the_Media_in_Nigeria

[3] Otana, Okinm-Alobi.Okpara, Ngozi. (2017, October). *Health Communication: The Responsibility of the Media in Nigeria*. ResearchGate. https://www.researchgate.net/publication/320265191_Health_Communication_The_Responsibility_of_the_Media_in_Nigeria

[4] Otana, Okinm-Alobi.Okpara, Ngozi. (2017, October). *Health Communication: The Responsibility of the Media in Nigeria*. ResearchGate. https://www.researchgate.net/publication/320265191_Health_Communication_The_Responsibility_of_the_Media_in_Nigeria

[5] Totomade, Samson. (2020, August 5). Former YPP presidential candidate Moghalu denies joining APC. *Pulse.ng*. https://www.pulse.ng/news/politics/ypps-moghalu-denies-joining-apc/79nn58r

[6] Somoye, Kehinde Gbolahan. (2015, May). Critical Review of the Management of Health Care System in Nigeria: Emphasis on Health Workforce. *International Journal of Scientific and Research Publications*. https://www.researchgate.net/publication/313163903_Critical_Review_of_the_Management_of_Health_Care_System_in_Nigeria_Emphasis_on_Health_Workforce

[7] Safari, Saeed; Baratloo, Alireza; Yousefifard, Mahmoud. (2015). Medical Journalism and Emergency Medicine. *National Center for Biotechnology Information*. https://www.ncbi.nlm.nih.gov/pmc/articles/PMC4608339/#B8

[8] Studholme, Liz. Traditional vs Digital Media: Which Should I Use in My Accounting or Bookkeeping Firm? *Boma*. https://bomamarketing.com/2018/06/24/traditional-vs-digital-media-which-should-i-use-in-my-business

[9] Mills, Ann. (2018, December 26). 5 MORE Signs Digital Marketing is Replacing Traditional Media. *ResourcefulBusiness*. https://resourcefulbusiness.com/5-more-signs-digital-marketing-is-replacing-traditional-media

[10] Statista. (2022). Percentage of population using the internet in Nigeria from 2000 to 2019. https://www.statista.com/statistics/643755/nigeria-internet-penetration.

[11] *Digital Content Publishers of Nigeria*. Publishersglobal.com. https://www.publishersglobal.com/directory/nigeria/media/digital-content-publishers

[12] *Reading:Advertising*. Lumen Principles of Marketing. https://courses.lumenlearning.com/clinton-marketing/chapter/reading-advertising

[13] Jibril, Ahmed Tanimu. (2017, September). *Reviewing the Concept of Advertising from the Print Media Perspectives*. Journal of Creative Communications. https://www.researchgate.net/publication/320040264_Reviewing_the_Concept_of_A dvertising_from_the_Print_Media_Perspectives

[14] Burstein, Daniel. (2017, May 2). Advertising Chart: Why customers ignore some newspaper and magazine ads. *MarketingSherpa*. https://www.marketingsherpa.com/article/chart/why-customers-ignore-some-print

[15] Oyama, Akim-Alobi. Okpara, Ngozi. (2017, October). Health Communication: The Responsibility of the Media in Nigeria. *Science Arena Publications Specialty Journal of Medical Research and Health Sciences*. https://www.researchgate.net/publication/320265191_Health_Communication_The_ Responsibility_of_the_Media_in_Nigeria

[16] Burstein, Daniel. (2017, May 2). Advertising Chart: Why customers ignore some newspaper and magazine ads. *MarketingSherpa*. https://www.marketingsherpa.com/article/chart/why-customers-ignore-some-print

[17] *First Case of Corona Virus Disease Confirmed in Nigeria*. (2020, February 28). Nigeria Centre for Disease Control. https://ncdc.gov.ng/news/227/first-case-of-corona-virus-disease-confirmed-in-nigeria

[18] *Nigeria's media landcape undergoes rapid change*. Oxford Business Group. https://oxfordbusinessgroup.com/overview/engaging-modern-audience-sector-undergoes-period-rapid-change

[19] *List of Nigerian magazines and journals*. W3newspapers. https://www.w3newspapers.com/nigeria/magazines

[20] Oloyede, Bayo I. Oni, Babatunde, O. Oluwole, Adefemi, V. (2015). Religion and media in a plural society: the Nigerian experience. *Raketa-production*. https://cyberleninka.ru/article/n/religion-and-media-in-a-plural-society-the-nigerian-experience/viewer

[21] Gerety, Rowan Moore. (2013, December 19). In Nigeria, Miracles Compete with Modern Medicine. *The Atlantic*. https://www.theatlantic.com/international/archive/2013/12/in-nigeria-miracles-compete-with-modern-medicine/282517

[22] *Media Landscapes*. Nigeria—Overview. Medialandscapes.com. https://medialandscapes.org/country/nigeria

[23] Idris, Abubakar. (2020, June 25). COVID-19 is quietly threatening the future of Nigeria's news media. *TechCabal*. https://techcabal.com/2020/06/25/covid-19-is-quietly-threatening-the-future-of-nigerias-news-media

[24] Akinwotu, Emmanuel. Burke, Jason. (2020, *April 4). Deaths in Nigerian city raise concerns over undetected Covid-19 outbreaks. The Guardian*. https://www.theguardian.com/world/2020/apr/28/nigerian-authorities-deny-wave-of-deaths-is-due-to-covid-19

[25] Oyekanmi, Samuel. (2021, November 10). COVID-10 Update in Nigeria. *Nairametrics*. https://nairametrics.com/2020/08/17/covid-19-update-in-nigeria

[26] US Department of Commerce. (1977, January 3*). Commerce America: Printing & Graphics Arts Equipment Catalog Exhibit, Lagos, Nigeria, June 6-10.* https://books.google.com/books?id=QSRei5b3QEwC

[27] Nwanguma, Uchechi Queen. (2015). *New Media and the Overlapping Roles of Content Providers and Content Consumers.* New Media and Mass Communications. (Vol. 41, 2015). *International Knowledge Sharing Platform.* https://www.iiste.org/Journals/index.php/NMMC/article/viewFile/25772/26099

[28] Wilding, Derek. Fray, Peter. (2018, October). The Impact of Digital Platforms on News and Journalism Content. *Center for Media Transition.* https://www.accc.gov.au/system/files/ACCC%20commissioned%20report%20-%20The%20impact%20of%20digital%20platforms%20on%20news%20and%20jour nalistic%20content%2C%20Centre%20for%20Media%20Transition%20%282%29. pdf

[29] *Reliefweb.* (2018, April 12). Health Ministry & WHO Train Health Journalists. https://reliefweb.int/report/nigeria/health-ministry-who-train-health-journalists

[30] *Reliefweb.* (2018, April 12). Health Ministry & WHO Train Health Journalists. https://reliefweb.int/report/nigeria/health-ministry-who-train-health-journalists

[31] Quinn, Katherine. (2017). Digital Media taken out Print Media. *Emerging Media 360.* (Loyola University, Maryland). https://www.loyola.edu/academics/emerging-media/blog/2017/digital-media-taken-out-print-media

[32] Nwanguma, Uchechi Queen. (2015). *New Media and the Overlapping Roles of Content Providers and Content Consumers.* New Media and Mass Communications. (Vol. 41, 2015). *International Knowledge Sharing Platform.* https://www.iiste.org/Journals/index.php/NMMC/article/viewFile/25772/26099

[33] Nwanguma, Uchechi Queen. (2015). *New Media and the Overlapping Roles of Content Providers and Content Consumers.* New Media and Mass Communications. (Vol. 41, 2015). *International Knowledge Sharing Platform.* https://www.iiste.org/Journals/index.php/NMMC/article/viewFile/25772/26099

Chapter Two

[1] Leask, Julie. Hooker, Claire. King, Catherine. (2010, September 8). Media coverage of health issues and how to work more effectively with journalists: a qualitative study. *BMC Public Health.* https://bmcpublichealth.biomedcentral.com/articles/10.1186/1471-2458-10-535

[2] Wakefield, Melanie A.; Loken, Barbara; Hornik, Robert C. (2010, October 9). Use of mass media campaigns to change health behaviour. *National Center for Biotechnology Information.* https://www.ncbi.nlm.nih.gov/pmc/articles/PMC4248563

3 *WaterAid*. Mass behavior change campaigns: What works and what doesn't. https://www.communityledtotalsanitation.org/sites/communityledtotalsanitation.org/files/Mass_behaviour_change_campaigns_briefing_note.pdf

4 *WaterAid*. Mass behavior change campaigns: What works and what doesn't. https://www.communityledtotalsanitation.org/sites/communityledtotalsanitation.org/files/Mass_behaviour_change_campaigns_briefing_note.pdf

5 Shrivastava, Saurabh R.; Shrivastava, Prateek S.; Ramasamy, Jeegadeesh. (2015, March 20). Public health strategies to ensure optimal community participation in the Ebola outbreak in West-Africa. *National Center for Biotechnology Information*. https://www.ncbi.nlm.nih.gov/pmc/articles/PMC4468240

6 Abroms, Lorien C.; Maibach, Edward W. (2008, January 3). The Effectiveness of Mass Communication to Change Public Behavior. *Annual Reviews*. https://www.annualreviews.org/doi/full/10.1146/annurev.publhealth.29.020907.090824

7 Wakefield, Melanie A.; Loken, Barbara; Hornik, Robert C. (2010, October 9). Use of mass media campaigns to change health behaviour. *National Center for Biotechnology Information*. https://www.ncbi.nlm.nih.gov/pmc/articles/PMC4248563

8 Abroms, Lorien C.; Maibach, Edward W. (2008, January 3). The Effectiveness of Mass Communication to Change Public Behavior. *Annual Reviews*. https://www.annualreviews.org/doi/full/10.1146/annurev.publhealth.29.020907.090824

9 Wakefield, Melanie A.; Loken, Barbara; Hornik, Robert C. (2010, October 9). Use of mass media campaigns to change health behaviour. *National Center for Biotechnology Information*. https://www.ncbi.nlm.nih.gov/pmc/articles/PMC4248563

10 Wakefield, Melanie A.; Loken, Barbara; Hornik, Robert C. (2010, October 9). Use of mass media campaigns to change health behaviour. *National Center for Biotechnology Information*. https://www.ncbi.nlm.nih.gov/pmc/articles/PMC4248563

11 Wakefield, Melanie A.; Loken, Barbara; Hornik, Robert C. (2010, October 9). Use of mass media campaigns to change health behaviour. *National Center for Biotechnology Information*. https://www.ncbi.nlm.nih.gov/pmc/articles/PMC4248563

12 Campbell, Christina. (2018, January 18). Failures of Nigerian Health Insurance Scheme: the way forward. *The Guardian*. https://guardian.ng/features/science/failures-of-nigerian-health-insurance-scheme-the-way-forward

13 Campbell, Christina. (2018, January 18). Failures of Nigerian Health Insurance Scheme: the way forward. *The Guardian*. https://guardian.ng/features/science/failures-of-nigerian-health-insurance-scheme-the-way-forward

[14] Wakefield, Melanie A.; Loken, Barbara; Hornik, Robert C. (2010, October 9). Use of mass media campaigns to change health behaviour. *National Center for Biotechnology Information.* https://www.ncbi.nlm.nih.gov/pmc/articles/PMC4248563

[15] Oladepo, Oladimeji; Oluwasanu, Mojisola; Abiona, Opeyemi. (2018). Analysis of tobacco control policies in Nigeria; historical development and application of multisectoral action. *BMC Public Health.* https://bmcpublichealth.biomedcentral.com/articles/10.1186/s12889-018-5831-9

[16] Wakefield, Melanie A.; Loken, Barbara; Hornik, Robert C. (2010, October 9). Use of mass media campaigns to change health behaviour. *National Center for Biotechnology Information.* https://www.ncbi.nlm.nih.gov/pmc/articles/PMC4248563

[17] Wakefield, Melanie A.; Loken, Barbara; Hornik, Robert C. (2010, October 9). Use of mass media campaigns to change health behaviour. *National Center for Biotechnology Information.* https://www.ncbi.nlm.nih.gov/pmc/articles/PMC4248563

[18] Shehu, R.A.; Namanya, S.A.; Ognibene, T.A.; Ogunsakin, E.A.; Baba, D.A. (2013, May 8). Lifestyle, fitness and health promotion initiative of the University of Ilorin, Nigeria: an educational media intervention. *American Journals Online.* Ethiopian Journal of Environmental Studies and Management, Vol. 6, No. 3, 2013. http://dx.doi.org/10.4314/ejesm.v6i3.7

[19] Mgbor, Michael O. (2006). Issues and Future Direction of Physical Education in Nigeria. *The Educational Forum.* https://files.eric.ed.gov/fulltext/EJ724646.pdf

[20] Mgbor, Michael O. (2006). Issues and Future Direction of Physical Education in Nigeria. *The Educational Forum.* https://files.eric.ed.gov/fulltext/EJ724646.pdf

[21] Wakefield, Melanie A.; Loken, Barbara; Hornik, Robert C. (2010, October 9). Use of mass media campaigns to change health behaviour. *National Center for Biotechnology Information.* https://www.ncbi.nlm.nih.gov/pmc/articles/PMC4248563

[22] Wakefield, Melanie A.; Loken, Barbara; Hornik, Robert C. (2010, October 9). Use of mass media campaigns to change health behaviour. *National Center for Biotechnology Information.* https://www.ncbi.nlm.nih.gov/pmc/articles/PMC4248563

[23] Brownson RC, Haire-Joshu D, Luke DA. Shaping the context of health: a review of environmental and policy approaches in the prevention of chronic diseases. *Annu Rev Public Health.* 2006;27:341–70. https://www.annualreviews.org/doi/pdf/10.1146/annurev.publhealth.27.021405.102137

[24] Wakefield, Melanie A.; Loken, Barbara; Hornik, Robert C. (2010, October 9). Use of mass media campaigns to change health behaviour. *National Center for Biotechnology Information.* https://www.ncbi.nlm.nih.gov/pmc/articles/PMC4248563

25 *World Health Organization.* (2007). Prevention of Cardiovascular Disease: Guidelines for assessment and management of cardiovascular risk. https://www.who.int/cardiovascular_diseases/guidelines/Full%20text.pdf

26 *World Health Organization.* (2007). Prevention of Cardiovascular Disease: Guidelines for assessment and management of cardiovascular risk. https://www.who.int/cardiovascular_diseases/guidelines/Full%20text.pdf

27 *World Health Organization.* (2007). Prevention of Cardiovascular Disease: Guidelines for assessment and management of cardiovascular risk. https://www.who.int/cardiovascular_diseases/guidelines/Full%20text.pdf

28 Wakefield, Melanie A.; Loken, Barbara; Hornik, Robert C. (2010, October 9). Use of mass media campaigns to change health behaviour. *National Center for Biotechnology Information.* https://www.ncbi.nlm.nih.gov/pmc/articles/PMC4248563

29 *World Health Organization.* (2007). Prevention of Cardiovascular Disease: Guidelines for assessment and management of cardiovascular risk. https://www.who.int/cardiovascular_diseases/guidelines/Full%20text.pdf

30 Welcome, Menizibeya Osain. (2011, October-December). The Nigerian health care system: Need for integrating adequate medical intelligence and surveillance systems. *National Center for Biotechnology Information.* https://www.ncbi.nlm.nih.gov/pmc/articles/PMC3249694

31 Okunola, Akindare. (2020, June 9). 5 Challenges Facing Health Care Workers in Nigeria as They Tackle COVID-19. *Global Citizen.* https://www.globalcitizen.org/en/content/challenges-for-health-care-workers-nigeria-covid

32 Gallagher, James. (2020, July 15). Fertility rate: 'Jaw-dropping' global crash in children being born. *BBC.* https://www.bbc.com/news/health-53409521#:~:text=In%201950%2C%20women%20were%20having,fall%20below%201.7%20by%202100

33 Wakefield, Melanie A.; Loken, Barbara; Hornik, Robert C. (2010, October 9). Use of mass media campaigns to change health behaviour. *National Center for Biotechnology Information.* https://www.ncbi.nlm.nih.gov/pmc/articles/PMC4248563

34 Wakefield, Melanie A.; Loken, Barbara; Hornik, Robert C. (2010, October 9). Use of mass media campaigns to change health behaviour. *National Center for Biotechnology Information.* https://www.ncbi.nlm.nih.gov/pmc/articles/PMC4248563

35 Wakefield, Melanie A.; Loken, Barbara; Hornik, Robert C. (2010, October 9). Use of mass media campaigns to change health behaviour. *National Center for Biotechnology Information.* https://www.ncbi.nlm.nih.gov/pmc/articles/PMC4248563

36 Wakefield, Melanie A.; Loken, Barbara; Hornik, Robert C. (2010, October 9). Use of mass media campaigns to change health behaviour. *National Center for*

Biotechnology Information.
https://www.ncbi.nlm.nih.gov/pmc/articles/PMC4248563

[37] Wakefield, Melanie A.; Loken, Barbara; Hornik, Robert C. (2010, October 9). Use of mass media campaigns to change health behaviour. *National Center for Biotechnology Information.*
https://www.ncbi.nlm.nih.gov/pmc/articles/PMC4248563

[38] Wakefield, Melanie A.; Loken, Barbara; Hornik, Robert C. (2010, October 9). Use of mass media campaigns to change health behaviour. *National Center for Biotechnology Information.*
https://www.ncbi.nlm.nih.gov/pmc/articles/PMC4248563

[39] Ogunbode, O.O., Ayinda, O.A. (2006, June 23). Awareness of cervical cancer and screening in a Nigerian female market population. *Annals of African Medicine.*
https://www.ajol.info/index.php/aam/article/view/8354

[40] Ogunbode, O.O., Ayinda, O.A. (2006, June 23). Awareness of cervical cancer and screening in a Nigerian female market population. *Annals of African Medicine.*
https://www.ajol.info/index.php/aam/article/view/8354

[41] Wakefield, Melanie A.; Loken, Barbara; Hornik, Robert C. (2010, October 9). Use of mass media campaigns to change health behaviour. *National Center for Biotechnology Information.*
https://www.ncbi.nlm.nih.gov/pmc/articles/PMC4248563

[42] Hill, David., Marks, Robin. (2008, April). Health promotion programs for melanoma prevention: screw or spring? *National Center for Biotechnology Information.*
https://pubmed.ncbi.nlm.nih.gov/18427051

[43] Hill, David., Marks, Robin. (2008, April). Health promotion programs for melanoma prevention: screw or spring? *National Center for Biotechnology Information.*
https://pubmed.ncbi.nlm.nih.gov/18427051

[44] *World Health Organization.* Regional Office for the Eastern Mediterranean. (2006). Guidelines for the early detection and screening of breast cancer: quick reference guide. https://apps.who.int/iris/handle/10665/119811

[45] Bello, Motunrayo. (2012, March 1). Awareness is the first step in battle against breast cancer. *National Center for Biotechnology Information.* DOI: 10.2471/BLT.12.030312. https://pubmed.ncbi.nlm.nih.gov/22461709

[46] Wakefield, Melanie A.; Loken, Barbara; Hornik, Robert C. (2010, October 9). Use of mass media campaigns to change health behaviour. *National Center for Biotechnology Information.*
https://www.ncbi.nlm.nih.gov/pmc/articles/PMC4248563

[47] Olasehinde, Olalekan; Boutin-Foster, Carla; Alatise, Lousegun I.; Adisa, Adewale O.; Lawal, Oladejo O.; Akinkuolie, Akinbolaji A.; Adesunkanmi, Abdul-Rasheed K.; Arije, Olujide O.; Kingham, Thomas P. (2017, January 25). Developing a Breast Cancer Screening Program in Nigeria: Evaluating Current Practices, Perceptions, and Possible Barriers. *National Center for Biotechnology Information.*
https://www.ncbi.nlm.nih.gov/pmc/articles/PMC5646896

⁴⁸ *World Health Organization.* (2014). WHO Position Paper on Mammography Screening. https://www.ncbi.nlm.nih.gov/books/NBK269535

⁴⁹ *World Health Organization.* WHO Position Paper on Mammography Screening. https://paho.org/hq/dmdocuments/2015/WHO-ENG-Mammography-Factsheet.pdf

⁵⁰ Wakefield, Melanie A.; Loken, Barbara; Hornik, Robert C. (2010, October 9). Use of mass media campaigns to change health behaviour. *National Center for Biotechnology Information.* https://www.ncbi.nlm.nih.gov/pmc/articles/PMC4248563

⁵¹ *Cancer Council.* (2019, December 2). Bowel cancer campaigns could save over 4300 Australian lives. https://www.cancer.org.au/media-releases/2019/bowel-cancer-campaigns-could-save-over-4300-australian-lives

⁵² Onyekwere, Charles A.; Ogbera, Anthonia O.; Abdulkareem, Fatima B.; Ashindoitiang, John. (2009, January 20). Colorectal Carinoma Screening in Lagos, Nigeria, Are We Doing it Right? *National Center for Biotechnology Information.* https://www.ncbi.nlm.nih.gov/pmc/articles/PMC5139884

⁵³ Onyekwere, Charles A.; Ogbera, Anthonia O.; Abdulkareem, Fatima B.; Ashindoitiang, John. (2009, January 20). Colorectal Carinoma Screening in Lagos, Nigeria, Are We Doing it Right? *National Center for Biotechnology Information.* https://www.ncbi.nlm.nih.gov/pmc/articles/PMC5139884

⁵⁴ Wakefield, Melanie A.; Loken, Barbara; Hornik, Robert C. (2010, October 9). Use of mass media campaigns to change health behaviour. *National Center for Biotechnology Information.* https://www.ncbi.nlm.nih.gov/pmc/articles/PMC4248563

⁵⁵ Hill, David., Marks, Robin. (2008, April). Health promotion programs for melanoma prevention: screw or spring? *National Center for Biotechnology Information.* https://pubmed.ncbi.nlm.nih.gov/18427051

⁵⁶ Wakefield, Melanie A.; Loken, Barbara; Hornik, Robert C. (2010, October 9). Use of mass media campaigns to change health behaviour. *National Center for Biotechnology Information.* https://www.ncbi.nlm.nih.gov/pmc/articles/PMC4248563

⁵⁷ Wakefield, Melanie A.; Loken, Barbara; Hornik, Robert C. (2010, October 9). Use of mass media campaigns to change health behaviour. *National Center for Biotechnology Information.* https://www.ncbi.nlm.nih.gov/pmc/articles/PMC4248563

⁵⁸ *World Health Organization.* (2019, November 16). Nigeria launches campaign to protect more than 28 million children against Measles and Meningitis. https://www.afro.who.int/news/nigeria-launches-campaign-protect-more-28-million-children-against-measles-and-meningitis

⁵⁹ *Google.* Diarrhea Disease Prevention. https://www.google.com/search?q=Diarrhea+Disease+Prevention&rlz=1C1SQJL_en NG883NG883

⁶⁰ Wakefield, Melanie A.; Loken, Barbara; Hornik, Robert C. (2010, October 9). Use of mass media campaigns to change health behaviour. *National Center for*

Biotechnology Information.
https://www.ncbi.nlm.nih.gov/pmc/articles/PMC4248563

[61] Wakefield, Melanie A.; Loken, Barbara; Hornik, Robert C. (2010, October 9). Use of mass media campaigns to change health behaviour. *National Center for Biotechnology Information.*
https://www.ncbi.nlm.nih.gov/pmc/articles/PMC4248563

[62] *DefeatDD.* Oral Rehydration Solution (ORS) + Zinc Co-Pack.
https://www.defeatdd.org/ors-zinc-copack

[63] Omuemu, Vivian O.; Ofuani, Ifeanyi J.; Kubeyinje, Itse C. (2012, March 4) Knowledge and Use of Zinc Supplementation in the Management of Childhood Diarrhoea among Health Care Workers in Public Primary Health Facilities in Benin-City, Nigeria. *National Center for Biotechnology Information.*
https://www.ncbi.nlm.nih.gov/pmc/articles/PMC4777055

[64] Brieger, William. (1990, March). Mass media and health communication in rural Nigeria. *ResearchGate.*
https://www.researchgate.net/publication/31225366_Mass_media_and_health_comm unication_in_rural_Nigeria.

[65] Wakefield, Melanie A.; Loken, Barbara; Hornik, Robert C. (2010, October 9). Use of mass media campaigns to change health behaviour. *National Center for Biotechnology Information.*
https://www.ncbi.nlm.nih.gov/pmc/articles/PMC4248563

[66] Ogundipe, Sola; Obinna, Chioma. (2011, August 7). Exclusive breast feeding: Whither Nigeria in the campaign? *Vanguard.*
https://www.vanguardngr.com/2011/08/exclusive-breast-feeding-whither-nigeria-in-the-campaign

[67] Chukwu-Okoronkwo, Samuel Okoronkwo. (2019, July). Impact Assessment of Exclusive Breastfeeding Media Campaign Among Mothers in Selected Metropolitan Cities in South East Nigeria 1*. *ResearchGate.*
https://www.researchgate.net/publication/334867084_Impact_Assessment_of_Exclu sive_Breastfeeding_Media_Campaign_Among_Mothers_in_Selected_Metropolitan_ Cities_in_South_East_Nigeria_1

[68] Wakefield, Melanie A.; Loken, Barbara; Hornik, Robert C. (2010, October 9). Use of mass media campaigns to change health behaviour. *National Center for Biotechnology Information.*
https://www.ncbi.nlm.nih.gov/pmc/articles/PMC4248563

[69] Wakefield, Melanie A.; Loken, Barbara; Hornik, Robert C. (2010, October 9). Use of mass media campaigns to change health behaviour. *National Center for Biotechnology Information.*
https://www.ncbi.nlm.nih.gov/pmc/articles/PMC4248563

[70] Wakefield, Melanie A.; Loken, Barbara; Hornik, Robert C. (2010, October 9). Use of mass media campaigns to change health behaviour. *National Center for Biotechnology Information.*
https://www.ncbi.nlm.nih.gov/pmc/articles/PMC4248563

[71] Wakefield, Melanie A.; Loken, Barbara; Hornik, Robert C. (2010, October 9). Use of mass media campaigns to change health behaviour. *National Center for Biotechnology Information.*
https://www.ncbi.nlm.nih.gov/pmc/articles/PMC4248563

[72] *Global Alliance of NGOs for Road Safety.* (2015, August 28). Nigerian NGO Safety Beyond Borders reduces traffic crashes at night.
https://www.roadsafetyngos.org/events/nigerian-ngo-safety-beyond-borders-reduces-traffic-crashes-at-night

[73] *Global Alliance of NGOs for Road Safety.* (2015, August 28). Nigerian NGO Safety Beyond Borders reduces traffic crashes at night.
https://www.roadsafetyngos.org/events/nigerian-ngo-safety-beyond-borders-reduces-traffic-crashes-at-night

[74] *Global Alliance of NGOs for Road Safety.* (2015, August 28). Nigerian NGO Safety Beyond Borders reduces traffic crashes at night.
https://www.roadsafetyngos.org/events/nigerian-ngo-safety-beyond-borders-reduces-traffic-crashes-at-night

[75] *Global Alliance of NGOs for Road Safety.* (2015, August 28). Nigerian NGO Safety Beyond Borders reduces traffic crashes at night.
https://www.roadsafetyngos.org/events/nigerian-ngo-safety-beyond-borders-reduces-traffic-crashes-at-night

[76] Popoola, Ademola Alabi; Olanrewaju, Timothy Olusegun; Bolaji, Benjamin Olusomi; Ajiboye, Tajudeen Olalekan. (2018, October 26). Expanding renal transplantation organ donor pool in Nigeria. *Saudi Journal of Kidney Diseases and Transplantation.*
https://www.sjkdt.org/article.asp?issn=1319-2442;year=2018;volume=29;issue=5;spage=1181;epage=1187;aulast=Popoola

[77] Wakefield, Melanie A.; Loken, Barbara; Hornik, Robert C. (2010, October 9). Use of mass media campaigns to change health behaviour. *National Center for Biotechnology Information.*
https://www.ncbi.nlm.nih.gov/pmc/articles/PMC4248563

[78] Wakefield, Melanie A.; Loken, Barbara; Hornik, Robert C. (2010, October 9). Use of mass media campaigns to change health behaviour. *National Center for Biotechnology Information.*
https://www.ncbi.nlm.nih.gov/pmc/articles/PMC4248563

[79] Popoola, Ademola Alabi; Olanrewaju, Timothy Olusegun; Bolaji, Benjamin Olusomi; Ajiboye, Tajudeen Olalekan. (2018, October 26). Expanding renal transplantation organ donor pool in Nigeria. *Saudi Journal of Kidney Diseases and Transplantation.*
https://www.sjkdt.org/article.asp?issn=1319-2442;year=2018;volume=29;issue=5;spage=1181;epage=1187;aulast=Popoola

[80] Popoola, Ademola Alabi; Olanrewaju, Timothy Olusegun; Bolaji, Benjamin Olusomi; Ajiboye, Tajudeen Olalekan. (2018, October 26). Expanding renal transplantation organ donor pool in Nigeria. *Saudi Journal of Kidney Diseases and Transplantation.*
https://www.sjkdt.org/article.asp?issn=1319-2442;year=2018;volume=29;issue=5;spage=1181;epage=1187;aulast=Popoola

[81] Krug, Etienne G.; Dahlberg, Linda L.; Mercy, James A.; Zwi, Anthony B.; Lozano, Rafael. (2002). World report on violence and health. Geneva. *World Health Organization.* http://apps.who.int/iris/bitstream/handle/10665/42495/9241545615_eng.pdf;jsessioni d=D388221F7C0C454C419CA7344F1632FB?sequence=1

[82] Krug, Etienne G.; Dahlberg, Linda L.; Mercy, James A.; Zwi, Anthony B.; Lozano, Rafael. (2002). World report on violence and health. Geneva. *World Health Organization.* http://apps.who.int/iris/bitstream/handle/10665/42495/9241545615_eng.pdf;jsessioni d=D388221F7C0C454C419CA7344F1632FB?sequence=1

[83] Wakefield, Melanie A.; Loken, Barbara; Hornik, Robert C. (2010, October 9). Use of mass media campaigns to change health behaviour. *National Center for Biotechnology Information.* https://www.ncbi.nlm.nih.gov/pmc/articles/PMC4248563

[84] Wakefield, Melanie A.; Loken, Barbara; Hornik, Robert C. (2010, October 9). Use of mass media campaigns to change health behaviour. *National Center for Biotechnology Information.* https://www.ncbi.nlm.nih.gov/pmc/articles/PMC4248563

[85] Wakefield, Melanie A.; Loken, Barbara; Hornik, Robert C. (2010, October 9). Use of mass media campaigns to change health behaviour. *National Center for Biotechnology Information.* https://www.ncbi.nlm.nih.gov/pmc/articles/PMC4248563

[86] Krug, Etienne G.; Dahlberg, Linda L.; Mercy, James A.; Zwi, Anthony B.; Lozano, Rafael. (2002). World report on violence and health. Geneva. *World Health Organization.* http://apps.who.int/iris/bitstream/handle/10665/42495/9241545615_eng.pdf;jsessioni d=D388221F7C0C454C419CA7344F1632FB?sequence=1

[87] Krug, Etienne G.; Dahlberg, Linda L.; Mercy, James A.; Zwi, Anthony B.; Lozano, Rafael. (2002). World report on violence and health. Geneva. *World Health Organization.* http://apps.who.int/iris/bitstream/handle/10665/42495/9241545615_eng.pdf;jsessioni d=D388221F7C0C454C419CA7344F1632FB?sequence=1

[88] *Nigeria Health Watch.* (2018, June 21). Confronting Nigeria's growing epidemic of heart disease. https://nigeriahealthwatch.com/confronting-nigerias-growing-epidemic-of-heart-disease

[89] Wakefield, Melanie A.; Loken, Barbara; Hornik, Robert C. (2010, October 9). Use of mass media campaigns to change health behaviour. *National Center for Biotechnology Information.* https://www.ncbi.nlm.nih.gov/pmc/articles/PMC4248563

[90] Wakefield, Melanie A.; Loken, Barbara; Hornik, Robert C. (2010, October 9). Use of mass media campaigns to change health behaviour. *National Center for Biotechnology Information.* https://www.ncbi.nlm.nih.gov/pmc/articles/PMC4248563

[91] *Nigeria Health Watch*. (2018, June 21). Confronting Nigeria's growing epidemic of heart disease. https://nigeriahealthwatch.com/confronting-nigerias-growing-epidemic-of-heart-disease

[92] *Nigeria Health Watch*. (2018, June 21). Confronting Nigeria's growing epidemic of heart disease. https://nigeriahealthwatch.com/confronting-nigerias-growing-epidemic-of-heart-disease

[93] Wakefield, Melanie A.; Loken, Barbara; Hornik, Robert C. (2010, October 9). Use of mass media campaigns to change health behaviour. *National Center for Biotechnology Information*. https://www.ncbi.nlm.nih.gov/pmc/articles/PMC4248563

[94] *PharmAccess Foundation*. (2015, March). Nigerian Health Sector: Market Study Report. https://www.rvo.nl/sites/default/files/Market_Study_Health_Nigeria.pdf

[95] Riman, Hodo B.; Akpan, Emmanuel S. (2012, May 11). Healthcare Financing and Health outcomes in Nigeria: A State Level Study using Multivariate Analysis. University of Calabar, Nigeria. *Munich Personal RePEc Archive*. https://core.ac.uk/download/pdf/211611728.pdf

[96] Onokerhoraye, Andrew Goodwin. (1976, November-December). A suggested framework for the provision of health facilities in Nigeria. *Social Science & Medicine*. https://www.sciencedirect.com/science/article/abs/pii/0037785676900263

[97] *World Health Organization*. (2017). Primary health care systems (PRIMASYS): case study from Nigeria. License: CC BY-NC-SA 3.0 IGO. https://www.who.int/alliance-hpsr/projects/alliancehpsr_nigeriaprimasys.pdf?ua=1

[98] *Institute of Medicine*. (2002). Speaking of Health: Assessing Health Communication Strategies for Diverse Populations. Washington, DC: The National Academies Press. https://doi.org/10.17226/10018. https://www.ncbi.nlm.nih.gov/books/NBK222234

[99] *World Health Organization*. (2018). Multisectoral and intersectoral action for improved health and well-being for all: mapping of the WHO European Region Governance for a sustainable future: improving health and well-being for all. https://www.euro.who.int/__data/assets/pdf_file/0005/371435/multisectoral-report-h1720-eng.pdf

[100] *World Health Organization*. (2018). Multisectoral and intersectoral action for improved health and well-being for all: mapping of the WHO European Region Governance for a sustainable future: improving health and well-being for all. https://www.euro.who.int/__data/assets/pdf_file/0005/371435/multisectoral-report-h1720-eng.pdf

[101] *World Health Organization*. (2018). Multisectoral and intersectoral action for improved health and well-being for all: mapping of the WHO European Region Governance for a sustainable future: improving health and well-being for all. https://www.euro.who.int/__data/assets/pdf_file/0005/371435/multisectoral-report-h1720-eng.pdf

[102] *World Health Organization*. (2018). Multisectoral and intersectoral action for improved health and well-being for all: mapping of the WHO European Region Governance for a sustainable future: improving health and well-being for all.

https://www.euro.who.int/__data/assets/pdf_file/0005/371435/multisectoral-report-h1720-eng.pdf

[103] Hallo De Wolf, Antenor; Toebes, Brigit. (2016, December). Assessing Private Sector Involvement in Health Care and Universal Health Coverage in Light of the Right to Health. *National Center for Biotechnology Information.* https://www.ncbi.nlm.nih.gov/pmc/articles/PMC5394993

[104] Hallo De Wolf, Antenor; Toebes, Brigit. (2016, December). Assessing Private Sector Involvement in Health Care and Universal Health Coverage in Light of the Right to Health. *National Center for Biotechnology Information.* https://www.ncbi.nlm.nih.gov/pmc/articles/PMC5394993

[105] Hallo De Wolf, Antenor; Toebes, Brigit. (2016, December). Assessing Private Sector Involvement in Health Care and Universal Health Coverage in Light of the Right to Health. *National Center for Biotechnology Information.* https://www.ncbi.nlm.nih.gov/pmc/articles/PMC5394993

[106] Gandolf, Stewart. How to Define Your Target Audience – A Critical Health Care Marketing Success Factor. *Healthcare Success.* https://healthcaresuccess.com/blog/branding/define-target-audience.html

[107] Gandolf, Stewart. How to Define Your Target Audience – A Critical Health Care Marketing Success Factor. *Healthcare Success.* https://healthcaresuccess.com/blog/branding/define-target-audience.html

[108] Patel, Sujan. (2017, June 14). Customer Testimonials: 9 Content Strategies for Success. *Content Marketing Institute.* https://contentmarketinginstitute.com/2017/06/strategies-customer-testimonials-content

Chapter Three

[1] Changkija, Monalisa. (2020, November 16). Role of Media during the COVID-19 Pandemic & its Impact on Media. *The Morung Express.* https://morungexpress.com/role-of-media-during-the-covid-19-pandemic-its-impact-on-media

[2] *Communications Theory.* Functions of Mass Communication in Mass Communication. https://www.communicationtheory.org/functions-of-mass-communication/#:~:text=1)%20Surveillance%20of%20the%20Environment,informa tion%20to%20the%20human%20society.&text=are%20influenced%20to%20an%20 extent,in%20their%20discussions%20and%20

[3] *Communications Theory.* Functions of Mass Communication in Mass Communication. https://www.communicationtheory.org/functions-of-mass-communication/#:~:text=1)%20Surveillance%20of%20the%20Environment,informa tion%20to%20the%20human%20society.&text=are%20influenced%20to%20an%20 extent,in%20their%20discussions%20and%20

[4] *American Press Institute.* (2016, April 17). A new understanding: What makes people trust and rely on news.
https://www.americanpressinstitute.org/publications/reports/survey-research/trust-news/single-page

[5] *American Press Institute.* (2016, April 17). A new understanding: What makes people trust and rely on news.
https://www.americanpressinstitute.org/publications/reports/survey-research/trust-news/single-page

[6] *American Press Institute.* (2016, April 17). A new understanding: What makes people trust and rely on news.
https://www.americanpressinstitute.org/publications/reports/survey-research/trust-news/single-page

[7] Strömbäck, Jesper; Tsfati, Yari; Boomgaarden, Hajo; Damstra, Alyt; Lindgren, Elina; Vliegentart, Rens; Lindholm, Torun. (2020, April 24). News media trust and its impact on media use: toward a framework for future research. *Annals of the international Communication Association.* 44:2, 139-156, DOI: 10.1080/23808985.2020.1755338.
https://www.tandfonline.com/doi/full/10.1080/23808985.2020.1755338

[8] Obukoadata, Presly. (2014, December). Media surveillance function within the context of the Ebola outbreak in Nigeria: Influences and perceptual frames. International Journal of Scientific Research and Innovative Technology, Vol. 1 No. 5, pp. 53-66. *Researchgate.*
https://www.researchgate.net/publication/273760818_Media_surveillance_function_within_the_context_of_the_Ebola_outbreak_in_Nigeria_Influences_and_perceptual_frames_International_Journal_of_Scientific_Research_and_Innovative_Technology_Vol_1_No_5_pp_53

[9] Obukoadata, Presly. (2014, December). Media surveillance function within the context of the Ebola outbreak in Nigeria: Influences and perceptual frames. International Journal of Scientific Research and Innovative Technology, Vol. 1 No. 5, pp. 53-66. *Researchgate.*
https://www.researchgate.net/publication/273760818_Media_surveillance_function_within_the_context_of_the_Ebola_outbreak_in_Nigeria_Influences_and_perceptual_frames_International_Journal_of_Scientific_Research_and_Innovative_Technology_Vol_1_No_5_pp_53

[10] *Google.* EVD disease.
https://www.google.com/search?rlz=1C1SQJL_enNG883NG883&sxsrf=ALeKk02dsDBBl2EGGuHRVSTb11e8sslTcQ:1611659926310&q=evd+disease&sa=X&ved=2ahUKEwi67J-LvbnuAhVDqHEKHQR8DA8Q1QIoAXoECBIQAg&biw=1137&bih=543

[11] Shoemaker, Pamela J.; Vos, Timothy P. (2009, April 28). Gatekeeping Theory. *Routledge.* https://www.routledge.com/Gatekeeping-Theory/Shoemaker-Vos/p/book/9780415981392

[12] *Mass Communication Theory*. Gatekeeping Theory.
https://masscommtheory.com/theory-overviews/gatekeeping-theory

[13] Shoemaker, Pamela J.; Vos, Timothy P. (2009, April 28). Gatekeeping Theory.
Routledge. https://www.routledge.com/Gatekeeping-Theory/Shoemaker-
Vos/p/book/9780415981392

[14] Anonymous. (2012). A Primer on Communication studies. *LardBucket*.
https://2012books.lardbucket.org/books/a-primer-on-communication-
studies/index.html

[15] Anonymous. (2012). A Primer on Communication studies. *LardBucket*.
https://2012books.lardbucket.org/books/a-primer-on-communication-
studies/index.html

[16] Anonymous. (2012). A Primer on Communication studies. *LardBucket*.
https://2012books.lardbucket.org/books/a-primer-on-communication-
studies/index.html

[17] Anonymous. (2012). A Primer on Communication studies. *LardBucket*.
https://2012books.lardbucket.org/books/a-primer-on-communication-
studies/index.html

[18] Anonymous. (2012). A Primer on Communication studies. *LardBucket*.
https://2012books.lardbucket.org/books/a-primer-on-communication-
studies/index.html

[19] *National Center for Biotechnology Information*. (2013). The Future of the Public's
Health in the 21st Century. https://www.ncbi.nlm.nih.gov/books/NBK221227

[20] *National Center for Biotechnology Information*. (2013). The Future of the Public's
Health in the 21st Century. https://www.ncbi.nlm.nih.gov/books/NBK221227

[21] Schwitzer, Gary; Mudur, Ganapati; Henry, David; Wilson, Amanda; Goozner, Merrill;
Simbra, Maria; Sweet, Melissa; Baverstock, Katherine A. (2005, July 26). What Are
the Roles and Responsibilities of the Media in Disseminating Health Information?
Plos Medicine.
https://journals.plos.org/plosmedicine/article?id=10.1371/journal.pmed.0020215

[22] Bishwajit, Ghose. (2016, January). Role of Health Journalism in Promoting
Communication among Stakeholders in Healthcare Sector. *Researchgate*.
https://www.researchgate.net/publication/305643899_Role_of_Health_Journalism_i
n_Promoting_Communication_among_Stakeholders_in_Healthcare_Sector

[23] Schwitzer, Gary; Mudur, Ganapati; Henry, David; Wilson, Amanda; Goozner, Merrill;
Simbra, Maria; Sweet, Melissa; Baverstock, Katherine A. (2005, July 26). What Are
the Roles and Responsibilities of the Media in Disseminating Health Information?
Plos Medicine.
https://journals.plos.org/plosmedicine/article?id=10.1371/journal.pmed.0020215

[24] Bishwajit, Ghose. (2016, January). Role of Health Journalism in Promoting
Communication among Stakeholders in Healthcare Sector. *Researchgate*.
https://www.researchgate.net/publication/305643899_Role_of_Health_Journalism_i
n_Promoting_Communication_among_Stakeholders_in_Healthcare_Sector

[25] Bishwajit, Ghose. (2016, January). Role of Health Journalism in Promoting Communication among Stakeholders in Healthcare Sector. *Researchgate.* https://www.researchgate.net/publication/305643899_Role_of_Health_Journalism_i n_Promoting_Communication_among_Stakeholders_in_Healthcare_Sector

[26] *World Health Organization.* (2020, February 13). Supporting media to bust harmful myths on coronavirus disease. https://www.afro.who.int/news/supporting-media-bust-harmful-myths-coronavirus-disease

[27] *World Health Organization.* (2020, February 13). Supporting media to bust harmful myths on coronavirus disease. https://www.afro.who.int/news/supporting-media-bust-harmful-myths-coronavirus-disease

[28] *World Health Organization.* (2020, February 13). Supporting media to bust harmful myths on coronavirus disease. https://www.afro.who.int/news/supporting-media-bust-harmful-myths-coronavirus-disease

[29] *World Health Organization.* (2020, February 13). Supporting media to bust harmful myths on coronavirus disease. https://www.afro.who.int/news/supporting-media-bust-harmful-myths-coronavirus-disease

[30] Bishwajit G, José Y, Junior RP, et al. Role of Health Journalism in Promoting Communication among Stakeholders in Healthcare Sector: Scientific Foundation and Architecture. J Healthc Commun. 2016, 1:3. DOI: 10.4172/2472-1654.100016. https://www.primescholars.com/articles/role-of-health-journalism-in-promoting-communication-among-stakeholders-in-healthcare-sector-96200.html.

[31] *World Health Organization.* (2011). mHealth: New horizons for health through mobile technologies: second global survey on eHealth. https://www.who.int/goe/publications/goe_mhealth_web.pdf

[32] *World Health Organization.* (2011). mHealth: New horizons for health through mobile technologies: second global survey on eHealth. https://www.who.int/goe/publications/goe_mhealth_web.pdf

[33] *World Health Organization.* (2011). mHealth: New horizons for health through mobile technologies: second global survey on eHealth. https://www.who.int/goe/publications/goe_mhealth_web.pdf

[34] Schmeer, Kammi. Stakeholder Analysis Guidelines: Section 2. *World Health Organization: Workforce Alliance.* https://www.who.int/workforcealliance/knowledge/toolkit/33.pdf

[35] Bishwajit G, José Y, Junior RP, et al. Role of Health Journalism in Promoting Communication among Stakeholders in Healthcare Sector: Scientific Foundation and Architecture. J Healthc Commun. 2016, 1:3. DOI: 10.4172/2472-1654.100016. https://www.primescholars.com/articles/role-of-health-journalism-in-promoting-communication-among-stakeholders-in-healthcare-sector-96200.html

[36] Schmeer, Kammi. Stakeholder Analysis Guidelines: Section 2. *World Health Organization: Workforce Alliance.* https://www.who.int/workforcealliance/knowledge/toolkit/33.pdf

[37] Schmeer, Kammi. Stakeholder Analysis Guidelines: Section 2. *World Health Organization: Workforce Alliance.* https://www.who.int/workforcealliance/knowledge/toolkit/33.pdf

[38] Rouse, William B.; Serban, Nicoleta. (2014, July). Understanding and Managing the Complexity of Healthcare. *MIT Press.* https://mitpress.mit.edu/books/understanding-and-managing-complexity-healthcare

[39] Rouse, William B.; Serban, Nicoleta. (2014, July). *Understanding and Managing the Complexity of Healthcare. MIT Press.* https://mitpress.mit.edu/books/understanding-and-managing-complexity-healthcare

[40] Leask, Julie; Hooker, Claire; King, Catherine. (2010, September 8). Media coverage of health issues and how to work more effectively with journalists: a qualitative study. *BMC Public Health* **10,** 535 (2010). https://doi.org/10.1186/1471-2458-10-535

[41] Leask, Julie; Hooker, Claire; King, Catherine. (2010, September 8). Media coverage of health issues and how to work more effectively with journalists: a qualitative study. *BMC Public Health* **10,** 535 (2010). https://doi.org/10.1186/1471-2458-10-535

[42] *Inter Pres Service.* IPS capacity building empowers journalists. http://www.ipsnews.net/ips-capacity-building-knowledge-sharing-and-communicating-for-change-workshops-in-201617

[43] *World Health Organization.* WHO Strategic Communications Framework for effective communications. https://www.who.int/mediacentre/communication-framework.pdf

[44] *World Health Organization.* WHO Strategic Communications Framework for effective communications. https://www.who.int/mediacentre/communication-framework.pdf

[45] Bishwajit G, José Y, Junior RP, et al. Role of Health Journalism in Promoting Communication among Stakeholders in Healthcare Sector: Scientific Foundation and Architecture. J Healthc Commun. 2016, 1:3. DOI: 10.4172/2472-1654.100016. https://www.primescholars.com/articles/role-of-health-journalism-in-promoting-communication-among-stakeholders-in-healthcare-sector-96200.html

[46] Stephens, Stephanie. (2019, February 19). Medical Conferences: 'Should I Stay or Should I Go?' *Health eCareers.* https://www.healthecareers.com/article/medical-conferences-benefits-to-going

[47] Stephens, Stephanie. (2019, February 19). Medical Conferences: 'Should I Stay or Should I Go?' *Health eCareers.* https://www.healthecareers.com/article/medical-conferences-benefits-to-going

[48] Shuchman, Miriam. (2002, February 13). Journalists as Change Agents in Medicine and Health Care. *JAMA-Journal of the American Medical Association.* DOI: 10.1001/jama.287.6.776. https://jamanetwork.com/journals/jama/fullarticle/1844976

[49] Shuchman, Miriam. (2002, February 13). Journalists as Change Agents in Medicine and Health Care. *JAMA-Journal of the American Medical Association.* DOI: 10.1001/jama.287.6.776. https://jamanetwork.com/journals/jama/fullarticle/1844976

[50] *World Health Organization.* (2020, February 3). 2019 Novel Coronavirus (2019-nCoV): Strategic Preparedness and Response Plan. (2020, February 3). https://www.who.int/docs/default-source/coronavirus/srp-04022020.pdf

[51] *World Health Organization.* (2020, February 3). 2019 Novel Coronavirus (2019-nCoV): Strategic Preparedness and Response Plan. (2020, February 3). https://www.who.int/docs/default-source/coronaviruse/srp-04022020.pdf

[52] *World Health Organization.* (2020, February 3). 2019 Novel Coronavirus (2019-nCoV): Strategic Preparedness and Response Plan. (2020, February 3). https://www.who.int/docs/default-source/coronaviruse/srp-04022020.pdf

[53] Almaghlooth, Abdulla. (2013). The Relevance of Gatekeeping in the Process of Contemporary News Creation and Circulation in Saudi Arabia. *University of Salford School of Arts and Media.* https://usir.salford.ac.uk/id/eprint/31958/3/Final_thesis_Abdullah_Almaghlooth_june152014.pdf

[54] Almaghlooth, Abdulla. (2013). The Relevance of Gatekeeping in the Process of Contemporary News Creation and Circulation in Saudi Arabia. *University of Salford School of Arts and Media.* https://usir.salford.ac.uk/id/eprint/31958/3/Final_thesis_Abdullah_Almaghlooth_june152014.pdf

[55] Almaghlooth, Abdulla. (2013). The Relevance of Gatekeeping in the Process of Contemporary News Creation and Circulation in Saudi Arabia. *University of Salford School of Arts and Media.* https://usir.salford.ac.uk/id/eprint/31958/3/Final_thesis_Abdullah_Almaghlooth_june152014.pdf

[56] Amodu, Lanre; Usaini, Suleimanu; Ige, Oyinkansola. (2014, January). The Media as Fourth Estate of the Realm. *Department of International Relations and Political Science, Covenant University,* Ota. DOI: 10.13140/RG.2.2.19311.02720. https://www.researchgate.net/publication/308120682_The_Media_as_Fourth_Estate_of_the_Realm

[57] Changkija, Monalisa. (2020, November 16). Role of Media during the COVID-19 Pandemic & its Impact on Media. *The Morung Express.* https://morungexpress.com/role-of-media-during-the-covid-19-pandemic-its-impact-on-media

[58] Srivastava, Shilpa; Pant, Millie; Abraham, Ajith; Agrawal, Namrata. (2015, June 3). The Technological Growth in eHealth Services. *National Center for Biotechnology Information.* DOI: 10.1155/2015/894171. https://www.ncbi.nlm.nih.gov/pmc/articles/PMC4469784

[59] Srivastava, Shilpa; Pant, Millie; Abraham, Ajith; Agrawal, Namrata. (2015, June 3). The Technological Growth in eHealth Services. *National Center for Biotechnology Information.* DOI: 10.1155/2015/894171. https://www.ncbi.nlm.nih.gov/pmc/articles/PMC4469784

[60] Dutta, Mohan J.; Kaur-Gill, Satveer; Tan, Naomi; Lam, Chervin. (2018) mHealth, Health, and Mobility: A Culture-Centered Interrogation. In: Baulch E., Watkins J., Tariq A. (eds) mHealth Innovation in Asia. Mobile Communication in Asia: Local Insights, Global Implications. Springer, Dordrecht.

https://doi.org/10.1007/978-94-024-1251-2_6.
https://link.springer.com/chapter/10.1007/978-94-024-1251-2_6

[61] Dutta, Mohan J.; Kaur-Gill, Satveer; Tan, Naomi; Lam, Chervin. (2018) mHealth, Health, and Mobility: A Culture-Centered Interrogation. In: Baulch E., Watkins J., Tariq A. (eds) mHealth Innovation in Asia. Mobile Communication in Asia: Local Insights, Global Implications. Springer, Dordrecht. https://doi.org/10.1007/978-94-024-1251-2_6.
https://link.springer.com/chapter/10.1007/978-94-024-1251-2_6

[62] Dutta, Mohan J.; Kaur-Gill, Satveer; Tan, Naomi; Lam, Chervin. (2018) mHealth, Health, and Mobility: A Culture-Centered Interrogation. In: Baulch E., Watkins J., Tariq A. (eds) mHealth Innovation in Asia. Mobile Communication in Asia: Local Insights, Global Implications. Springer, Dordrecht. https://doi.org/10.1007/978-94-024-1251-2_6.
https://link.springer.com/chapter/10.1007/978-94-024-1251-2_6